"CEOs and board members will find *Getting to Great* practical and inspirational. This book is grounded in reality; it provides 'bite-size' and thought-provoking steps which, if taken, will enhance board, CEO, and organizational performance."
— Donald C. Sibery, president and CEO, and Steven V. Wilkinson,
   chair of the board of directors, Central DuPage Health, Winfield, Illinois

"This is the most practical and useful book on governance I have ever read. It boldly challenges boards and CEOS to transform the way governance is practiced in health care organizations."
— David J. Campbell, president and CEO, Saint Vincent
   Catholic Medical Centers of New York

"Pointer and Orlikoff present seventy-two implementable principles—useful for both new and long-tenured board members—for improving health care organization trusteeship."
— David J. Fine, president and CEO, UAB Health System, Birmingham, Alabama

"*Getting to Great* conveys a timely and timeless construct that will resonate with anyone looking for guidance to exercise governance responsibilities according to a prescription for excellence. Whether an organization is absorbed in a turnaround or has achieved peak performance, the principle-based governance model provides a template that will align management and board to accelerate the former and enhance the latter."
— Joseph R. Swedish, president and CEO, and P. Terrence O'Rourke,
   chairman of the board, Centura Health, Englewood, Colorado

"*Getting to Great* is one of the very best books written about a critical issue in health care governance. It is a must-read for CEOs and board members and comes along at just the right time. I highly recommend it.
— Charles S. Lauer, publisher, *Modern Healthcare,* and corporate vice president,
   Crain Communications, Inc.

"*Getting to Great* sets forth principles for dramatically improving board performance that are both conceptually sound and practical. Its guidance is forged from the authors' vast experience working with hundreds of health care organizations, and is conveyed with remarkable clarity and directness."
— William Dowling, professor and chair, Department of Health Services,
   School of Public Health and Community Medicine, University of Washington,
   Seattle, Washington

Getting to Great

Getting to Great

Principles of Health Care Organization Governance

Dennis D. Pointer
James E. Orlikoff

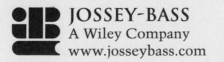
JOSSEY-BASS
A Wiley Company
www.josseybass.com

Published by

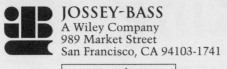

JOSSEY-BASS
A Wiley Company
989 Market Street
San Francisco, CA 94103-1741

www.josseybass.com

This publication is designed to provide accurate and authoritative information in regard to the subject matter covered. It is sold with the understanding that the publisher is not engaged in rendering professional services. If professional advice or other expert assistance is required, the services of a competent professional person should be sought.

Jossey-Bass books and products are available through most bookstores. To contact Jossey-Bass directly, call (888) 378-2537, fax to (800) 605-2665, or visit our website at www.josseybass.com.

Substantial discounts on bulk quantities of Jossey-Bass books are available to corporations, professional associations, and other organizations. For details and discount information, contact the special sales department at Jossey-Bass.

We at Jossey-Bass strive to use the most environmentally sensitive paper stocks available to us. Our publications are printed on acid-free recycled stock whenever possible, and our paper always meets or exceeds minimum GPO and EPA requirements.

Jossey-Bass also publishes its books in a variety of electronic formats. Some content that appears in print may not be available in electronic books.

Library of Congress Cataloging-in-Publication Data

Pointer, Dennis Dale.
  Getting to great/principles of health care organization governance/Dennis D. Pointer, James E. Orlikoff.
    p. cm.
  Includes bibliographical references and index.
  ISBN 0-7879-6121-3 (alk. paper)
    1. Introduction—Administration. 2. Health Facilities—Administration. 3. Hospital trustees. 4. Health Facilities—organization. 5. Governing board—organization & administration. I. Title. II. Orlikoff, James E.
  RA971 .P628   2002
  362.1'1'068—dc21   2002003291

HC Printing   10 9 8 7 6 5 4 3 2   FIRST EDITION

CONTENTS

THE AUTHORS

Dennis Pointer and James Orlikoff are among the nation's most highly regarded health care governance consultants, speakers, and writers. They have collaborated on two previous books published by Jossey-Bass: *Board Work: Governing Health Care Organizations,* winner of the James A. Hamilton Book of the Year Award from the American College of Healthcare Executives, and *The High-Performance Board: Principles of Nonprofit Organization Governance.*

Dennis D. Pointer has worked with over 450 clients. His firm, Dennis D. Pointer & Associates, provides governance consulting, retreat facilitation, assessment, redesign, and development services to health care organizations, other nonprofits, commercial corporations, and governmental agencies. He is vice president of the American Governance & Leadership Group, LLC. The author of six previous books and more than seventy articles, Dr. Pointer is Austin Ross Professor, Department of Health Services, School of Public Health and Community Medicine, University of Washington (Seattle). He has held two previous endowed chairs: the John J. Hanlon Professorship of Health Management and Policy, Graduate School of Public Health, San Diego State University; and the Arthur Graham Glasgow Chair, Department of Health Administration, Medical College of Virginia. From 1975 to 1986 he was affiliated with the University of California—Los Angeles, where he served as associate director of the UCLA Medical Center and as a professor in the Department of Health Services Management, School of Public Health, and also as its chair. While at UCLA, Pointer was a senior research fellow at RAND Corporation. He received his bachelor of science degree from Iowa State University and his doctorate from the University of Iowa.

James E. (Jamie) Orlikoff is president of Orlikoff & Associates, Inc., specializing in governance improvement and leadership development. He is executive director of the American Governance & Leadership Group, LLC, which provides educational conferences, on-site programs, and consulting services for boards, board members, and other health care leaders. Orlikoff is the national adviser on governance and leadership for the American Hospital Association and the former director of its Hospital Governance division. Orlikoff has worked with more than six hundred organizations to strengthen their governance effectiveness. He is the author of fourteen books and more than one hundred articles and is consulting editor for *American Governance Leader,* a monthly newsletter on leadership issues and trends for health care organization board members. Orlikoff received his bachelor of arts degree from Pitzer College in Claremont, California, and his master of arts degree from the University of Chicago. He currently serves on the Pitzer College board.

American Governance & Leadership Group (AG&L Group) is a partnership of the American Hospital Association, governance expert James E. Orlikoff, and educational developer Jerry F. Pogue. They are joined in this partnership by governance authorities Mary K. Totten and Dennis D. Pointer. AG&L Group is an educational resource for hospital and health system leaders, health care trustees, and physician group leaders. For information contact: *Info@AmericanGovernance.com* or (909) 336-1586.

Getting to Great

CHAPTER 1

Introduction

G overnance is important work. How well it is done has significant consequences for health care organizations, the communities they serve, and their patients, medical staffs, and employees.

Over the past twenty years, we have served on numerous boards, consulted with hundreds of boards, and written scores of books and articles about boards. We have a profound respect for the contributions they *can* make. Most boards truly want to make a difference and add value. The vast majority of board members are talented and committed individuals who devote incredible amounts of time and energy to governing. Yet performance of the typical health care organization board is far from optimal. The primary reason is that governance is often unfocused and idiosyncratic; it is not grounded on a coherent, precise, explicit "technology" and an associated set of principles that promote best practices and continuous improvement (see Box 1.1).

A *technology* is a set of principles for solving problems and seizing opportunities. Health care organization success depends on the quality of three of them:

- *Management technology:* Principles that help executives deploy an organization's resources in ways that accomplish goals
- *Clinical technology:* Principles that help medical professionals promote health, prevent disease, and provide caring and curing services to patients

- *Governance technology:* Principles that help boards effectively balance and represent the interests of stakeholders, to whom the organization "belongs"

Grounded on economics, sociology, and psychology, the discipline of management emerged after World War II. Taught in schools of business and conveyed in a vast literature, it incorporates a host of "subtechnologies" such as accounting and finance, strategy, marketing, operations design and management, human resources, and information systems.

Based on the biomedical model developed in the mid-1800s, modern clinical technology emerged in the early twentieth century; it has been refined and elaborated by a huge investment in basic and applied research over the past fifty years. The principles are taught in medical, nursing, and other health professional schools.

Managerial and clinical technologies are far more developed and sophisticated than the technology of governing. Yet a lot is known about boards and how they can more efficiently and effectively solve problems and seize opportunities in ways that enhance an organization's success.

Here is an example from the commercial sector. CalPERS, the California Public Employees Retirement System, is one of the largest pension funds in the country. In 1995–1996, it asked three hundred companies in its equity portfolio to consider adopting formal governance principles. CalPERS staff issued report cards, and a set of model principles were formulated and distributed. (You can see the latest version at http://www.calpers.org.) A Wilshire Associates study of the "CalPERS effect" examined the performance of sixty-two companies over a ten-year period. The results indicated that whereas the stock of these companies trailed the Standard & Poor's 500 Index by 89 percent during the five-year period before implementing CalPERS governance principles, they outperformed the S&P by 23 percent in the five years after adoption, contributing $150 million in additional value to the retirement fund annually.

About half the nation's largest commercial enterprises have adopted governance principles in some form (*Trustee Magazine,* July-Aug. 1998). Yet this is not common practice in health care organizations.

This book lays out a governance technology—a set of principles and associated practices based on a model of factors that most affect board performance and contributions. The principles are evidence-based, derived from our own consulting engagements, the governance literature, organization and management theory, and empirical research.

This book is written with a point-of-view and has an agenda. Because we believe that principle-based governance can dramatically enhance board performance and organizational success, our objective is to stimulate and facilitate the adoption of this approach in health care organizations. The book is targeted at board members and executives committed to improving governance practice (see Box 1.2). It is a book for serious people willing to make a significant investment in their board's and organization's future.

This is a practical, "how to" book; it provides

- A *model* of health care organization governance that serves as the framework for Chapters Three through Seven
- A set of seventy-two *governance principles* and associated practices for improving your board's performance and contributions

Box 1.2. Uses of This Book

- As a comprehensive *overview* of health care organization governance for newly appointed board members
- As a "best practice" *refresher* for experienced board members
- As an *exemplar* of what a truly great board should look like
- As a *blueprint* for transforming your board, designing and implementing specific principles and practices that will improve its performance and contributions
- As a *template* and a set of specific *criteria* for assessing governance quality

- *Getting-started recommendations* to help your board begin adopting the principles
- *Checkups* for assessing your board
- *Guidelines* for implementing principle-based governance

Charles Darwin observed that in challenging environments where resources are scarce, if an organism has even a tiny edge over others, this advantage is amplified over time. He noted, in *On the Origin of Species,* that a few grains of sand tip the balance, determining who thrives and who dies. Principle-based governance can tip a health care organization's balance toward success.

This book promotes an explicit, comprehensive, and coherent set of principles that set out what health care organization governance should look like at its very best. An executive summary is presented in Box 1.3.

As you read this book, you may begin to feel overwhelmed by the multitude of things your board can, and should, do to improve its performance and contributions. Our recommendation is, Don't be! Our approach to governance development can produce significant results when focused on implementing a *limited* set of principles; a "full court press," though perhaps ideal, is not necessary. This is a map for an entire journey that your board

Box 1.3. Executive Summary: Principles of Health Care Governance

The great board ...

- Appreciates the importance of governance and takes its work seriously
- Understands the factors that most affect governance quality and board performance
- Devotes the necessary time and effort to governing
- Governs on the basis of agreed-to and explicit principles

The great board meets its fiduciary obligations; it ...

- Identifies and prioritizes key stakeholders and understands their interests and expectations
- Represents stakeholders and ensures that the organization's resources and capacities are deployed in ways that benefit them
- Meets its fiduciary duties of loyalty and care

The great board fulfills its responsibility for organizational ends (destination); it ...

- Formulates a precise, detailed vision that defines what the organization should become, at its very best, in the future
- Specifies key organizational goals that must be accomplished for the vision to be fulfilled
- Ensures that management strategies are aligned with goals and the vision

The great board fulfills its responsibility for executive performance; it ...

- Specifies that the CEO is its *only* direct report
- Plans for CEO succession
- Undertakes an effective recruitment and selection process when the position of CEO becomes vacant

(Continued)

Box 1.3. Continued

- Specifies its expectations of the CEO
- Assesses the CEO's performance and provides him or her with feedback to improve it
- Adjusts the CEO's compensation based on an assessment of his or her performance
- Is prepared to terminate the CEO's employment, should the need arise

The great board fulfills its responsibility for quality; it . . .

- Develops an explicit and precise working definition of quality
- Credentials members of the medical staff and makes decisions regarding appointment, reappointment, and delineation of privileges
- Ensures that necessary quality and utilization management systems are in place and function effectively
- Assesses the quality of care provided in and by the organization
- Reviews management plans for managing, and continuously improving, quality and patient or customer satisfaction

The great board fulfills its responsibility for finances; it . . .

- Formulates key financial objectives
- Ensures that management-developed budgets lead to accomplishing financial objectives
- Assesses financial performance and outcomes
- Ensures that necessary financial controls are in place

The great board performs its core roles; it . . .

- Formulates policies that convey its expectations and directives
- Makes decisions regarding matters requiring its attention and input
- Monitors and assesses key organizational processes and outcomes

The great board is structured appropriately; it . . .

- Is streamlined, having the fewest possible layers of governance, boards, and committees
- Is the right size, having between eleven and nineteen members unless there is a compelling reason for a smaller or larger number of members
- Explicitly specifies the authority, responsibilities, and roles of multiple boards, if the organization has more than one
- Has the right number and types of committees to support and facilitate its work
- Precisely specifies its authority vis-à-vis committees, ensuring that the board governs and that committees perform governance "staff work"
- Specifies the objectives, functions, and tasks of its committees and requires that they develop annual work plans
- Reviews the performance of and need for every committee each year
- Periodically assesses the governance structure and modifies it when necessary

The great board has the right composition; it . . .

- Proactively designs and manages its own composition
- Recruits and selects new members on the basis of explicit criteria
- Has an effective new-member orientation process
- Specifies member expectations
- Has fixed member term lengths and limits
- Assesses the performance and contributions of individual members
- Ensures that members do not represent narrow interests or constituencies
- Includes the CEO as a voting member of the board
- Ensures that ex officio and "inside" members hold no more than 25 percent of the board's seats
- Periodically examines the assets and liabilities of compensating board members

(Continued)

The great board has the necessary infrastructure in place; it . . .

- Develops an annual governance budget
- Has adequate staff support
- Formulates annual governance objectives
- Employs a formal agenda planning and management process
- Ensures that board meetings are conducted in a way that maximizes their effectiveness, efficiency, and creativity
- Selects a chair that understands his or her role and is willing and able to perform it effectively
- Has a plan to continually develop board competencies and capacities
- Holds annual or semiannual retreats
- Undertakes periodic board self-assessment, employing the results to engage in action planning that improves governance quality

might want to take. Begin with the first steps, have modest initial goals, don't obsess on what's left to be done, celebrate wins, keep at it, and enjoy the trip!

Getting to Great is the product of what we have learned over the years from our fellow board members, clients, and consultant colleagues. They have been our teachers, and we are indebted to them.

We would be delighted to hear from you about your board's adventure of getting to great.

Dennis D. Pointer
Dennis D. Pointer & Associates
(206) 499–1289
www.benchmarkgovernance.com

James E. Orlikoff
Orlikoff & Associates, Inc.
(773) 268–8009
www.americangovernance.com

CHAPTER 2

Board and Governance Basics

A s John Carver observes in *Boards That Make a Difference*, boards are "as high up in organizations as one can go and still remain inside them." Accordingly, they bear ultimate authority and accountability for their organizations' affairs, what they are, and what they can become.

Governance is an activity, what boards do: serving as a trustee and steward of an organization's resources and capacities on behalf of those it is intended to benefit.

Boards govern as teams. Exercising collective influence, their members have no individual authority or power. Boards exist only when they meet, "between raps of the gavel." Members may disagree—they can and should debate and argue about issues; but to decide and act, they must do so together.

Governance is part-time and occasional work. While management, members of the medical staff, and employees are relatively permanent organizational fixtures, boards are not. They convene for a short period of time, they adjourn, and then weeks or months pass until they meet again. Their attention, time, and energy are limited and very fragmented. In addition, governance is a peripheral aspect of board members' lives. No matter how important the issues being addressed, they are pushed aside when meetings end.

We've come to three conclusions about governance.

First, governance really matters. A board has a significant impact on an organization's success or the lack thereof. Consider this challenge: Your board is given thirty minutes to make decisions that would cause the organization great harm. Could you do it? Most board members respond, "Absolutely. It would be easy, and our board would need only half the time." Does governance matter? You bet it does, for better or worse!

Second, governance is becoming more difficult. Due to the nature and pace of change taking place in the industry, increasing size and complexity of health care organizations and greater demands for accountability, the governance "cross bar" has been rising. More is being expected of boards (see Box 2.1).

Box 2.1. The Challenge of Governing

The nature of health care organization governance and what is being demanded of boards have changed dramatically. Here are two metaphors that capture and accentuate the differences between then and now.

Then: On an important journey, you come to a lake that must be crossed. A small boat is available; you get in and start rowing. Your destination is clearly visible. Planning and considerable energy will be required to get to where you want to go, but you have the necessary stamina and skills. The lake is calm, and the weather is not threatening. Occasionally, a storm appears, but it passes quickly and the lake returns to normal.

Now (and in the future): You're running a raging river through a steep canyon in a kayak. You can't plot the currents or see hidden rocks, and you don't know what's around the next bend. The risk of capsizing is great, and the consequences of doing so are serious. There are no patches of calm water where you can catch your breath; downstream are just more rapids.

Very different skills and a much higher level of metabolism are required to successfully kayak the rapids than to row across a calm lake!

Third, governance can dramatically improve organizational perform-ance. Boards can make more of a difference and add greater value. We have seen it happen. We have helped boards make it happen. But it does not happen fortuitously. Certain things are essential to improving gover-nance quality:

- Board members must be dissatisfied with the status quo. Boards that are pleased with their present level of performance do not change, as they see no need to do so.

- The board must have a clear image of what its governance can and should be like at its very best.

- Significant time and energy must be devoted to undertaking board development initiatives above and beyond what is already spent on governing.

- Continual follow-through and follow-up must keep the board on track. Major change always creates pressure for gradually returning to the more comfortable way things were done in the past.

To truly transform your board, its governance must be built on princi-ples that promote best practice. This book sets forth seventy-two govern-ing principles based on a model of factors that most affect board performance and contributions (see Figure 2.1). Here are definitions of terms as they are used in the figure and throughout this book:

- *Obligations:* the purpose of boards and their fiduciary duties
- *Functioning:* how boards define and fulfill their responsibilities and roles
- *Structure:* how governance work is subdivided, shared, and coordinated
- *Composition:* board member characteristics, knowledge, skills, experi-ence, and perspectives
- *Infrastructure:* governance enablers—resources and systems that sup-port boards and their work

Clearly, a host of factors affect governance quality. But these are the ones we have found to matter most. This prompts our first principle.

Figure 2.1. Key Determinants of Governance Performance and Contributions

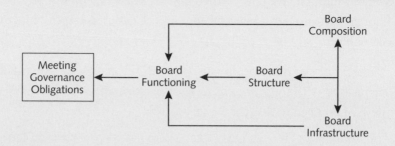

PRINCIPLE 1

The board realizes that it alone bears ultimate authority and accountability for the organization. It appreciates the importance of governance and undertakes its work with a sense of seriousness and purpose.

Your board has no capacity for doing the "real work" of the organization: providing patient care. Furthermore, it cannot manage the organization and should not attempt to do so. Yet it is ultimately responsible for both activities. Your board is, to paraphrase Harry Truman, where the buck stops.

Your board must appreciate its obligations if it is to fulfill them. Recognizing the importance of governance is a prerequisite for doing the job well. Few people are willing to devote time and effort to activities deemed insignificant.

We've worked with boards whose members believe governance is trivial, relatively inconsequential to the organization's success. We have worked with boards whose members are either unable or unwilling to devote the necessary time and energy to governing. In such cases, little can be done to improve governance practice; the motivation and energy necessary for doing so do not exist.

PRINCIPLE 2

The board understands the factors that most affect governance quality and employs a coherent set of principles to govern.

This is the fundamental principle behind this entire book.

Many boards practice idiosyncratic governance based largely on personal experience, situational logic, and habit. While this may yield acceptable and even occasionally good governance, it is an inherently limiting approach. Optimal board performance and contributions are based on principles that specify best practices regarding governance obligations, functions, structure, composition, and infrastructure.

Health care organizations and their boards are an extremely diverse lot. Some are large, multimarket enterprises having resources in the billions, rivaling those of Fortune 500 companies, with huge staffs. Wearing tailored suits, their members convene in specially designated board rooms and sit in leather chairs around walnut tables. Others are small, locally focused organizations with modest budgets and small staffs. Board members arrive wearing jeans and sweatshirts, and meetings are held in a staff conference room. When it comes to governing, these differences, though certainly noticeable, are superficial. All boards have identical obligations and must do the same type of work to meet them. And all boards must design their functioning, structure, composition, and infrastructure to perform this work well. Accordingly, there are generic and broadly applicable principles of governance that transcend an organization's characteristics and particular circumstances.

GOVERNANCE CHECKUP
Board Basics

Throughout the book, you will have the opportunity to examine your board. In Chapter Nine, your analyses will be combined to produce a governance profile. The Governance Checkups in each chapter are not comprehensive and should not be used to perform the kinds of thorough governance self-assessments we recommend in Principle 72. Rather, they have been designed to provide an initial "navigational fix" of the extent to which your board employs the principles promoted here.

When completing the Checkups, be descriptive and discriminating. Portray your board's actual characteristics and practices. Be honest and candid; don't fall victim to the "halo effect," giving everything high ratings. Most boards excel in some areas and not in others; your responses should reflect this.

Respond to all items.

	No	Not Entirely	Yes
1. My board appreciates the importance of governance to the organization, and takes its work seriously.	1	2	3
2. My board understand the factors that most affect its performance and contributions.	1	2	3
3. Members of my board devote the necessary time and effort to governing.	1	2	3
4. My board governs on the basis of an agreed set of explicit principles.	1	2	3

Total your responses for the four items, divide by 12, and then multiply by 100. The product is your board's percentage of the maximum score in this area.

Total _____ ÷ 12 × 100 = _____ percent

GETTING STARTED

✓ Continually reinforce the importance of the board and governance work: during the orientation of new members, through educational activities, at meetings, and before critical issues are addressed.

✓ Important work is appreciated, consistently and repeatedly. Seize every opportunity to acknowledge and celebrate your board's accomplishments and efforts.

✓ At an upcoming board meeting, hold a brief discussion focusing on your board's overall level of performance and contributions.

> How does your board rate?

> What are your board's greatest strengths and most significant weaknesses?

> What are some specific things your board could or should do to make more of a difference and add greater value?

✓ Begin crafting a few initial principles for your board, simple declarative statements that specify how it will govern.

✓ Employ the Getting Started checklists appearing throughout this book to begin formulating elements of a continuous improvement action plan for your board.

CHAPTER 3

Obligations

Why do boards exist? What is their purpose?

Your board has the potential to make a significant difference and add considerable value. But the key term is *potential*, which can be realized only if your board understands and fulfills its obligations.

PRINCIPLE 3

The overarching obligation of a board is ensuring that the organiza-tion's resources and capacities are deployed in ways that benefit stakeholders. The board is their agent; representing, protecting, and advancing their interests and acting on their behalf.

This principle goes to the heart of your board's fundamental purpose.

Every organization is intended to benefit someone. The question is who (see Box 3.1).

- Commercial corporations are formed to benefit *shareholders,* the people who own the corporations' stock.

- *Stakeholders* are the individuals and groups for the benefit of whom nonprofit organizations are created. They are the equivalent of the owners of a for-profit corporation. However, unlike shareholders, stakeholders are not actual owners and have no divisible claim on the organization's assets.

• Government agencies benefit *constituents:* voters, citizens, or the like.

When asked what a board's most fundamental and important obligation is, most board members respond, "We're here to look out for the organization, to ensure that it survives and thrives." This answer is off the mark and provides an inappropriate starting point for governing.

An organization is a collection of resources: money, people, facilities, equipment, supplies, and capabilities; it is a *means.* The *end* is benefiting stakeholders.

Your board's fundamental obligation is representing, advancing, and protecting the interests of stakeholders: making sure the organization benefits them; deciding and acting on their behalf; serving as their agent. Great (or even just good) governance begins with a clear, precise, and shared notion of the purpose for which your board exists. Only with clarity and consensus here can your board determine what it must do and how it should go about doing it.

PRINCIPLE 4

The board identifies the organization's key stakeholders.

Once your board understands its overarching obligation to stakeholders, it must identify them, explicitly and precisely (see Box 3.2).

It is here where health care organizations differ significantly from commercial corporations. The owners of commercial corporations are easily identified: everyone who owns stock.

Things are not so simple for health care organizations. Granted, the charter or articles of incorporation typically denote whom the organization was initially formed to benefit. However, the wording is usually quite vague. Phrases such as "the community," "the public," or "patients" are common.

So who are they? Some illustrative stakeholders are presented in Box 3.3.

Box 3.2. Stakeholders: Who Exactly Are They?

An easy question to answer, you say? Typically, that is *not* the case in most health care organizations.

When addressing this topic at board retreats, we ask members to take out a piece of paper and list their organization's most important stakeholders. Invariably, the responses are vague and there is not much agreement. Give this a try at your next board meeting.

How can your board fulfill its obligation to govern on behalf of stakeholders if members either do not know or disagree among themselves about who they are? The answer is, of course, that it cannot.

Box 3.3 Examples of Stakeholders in Various Organizations

Preferred Provider Organization

- Hospitals (who own class A stock)
- Hospitals (who own class B stock)
- Primary care physician members (who own class C stock)
- Primary care physician affiliates (who do not own stock)
- Specialty and subspecialty physician members (who own class C stock)
- Specialty and subspecialty physicians (who do not own stock)

Private College

- Students
- Parents of students
- Faculty
- Major donors
- The largest research funders
- Alumni

Professional Association

- Members who have attained fellowship status
- Members who are diplomates and associates
- Student affiliates
- Sponsoring organizations ("incorporators") named in the charter
- State agencies that license members of the profession
- "The public" (clients) who use services provided by members of the profession

Symphony Orchestra

- Corporate patrons
- Individual patrons
- Season ticket holders
- Regular event attendees

- Orchestra members
- City arts council

Faith-Based Short-Term General Hospital

- The sponsoring religious congregation
- The archdiocese
- Community benefit organizations in the primary service area that complement and support the hospital's mission
- Actual and potential patients and their families
- The poor and uninsured residing in the hospital's primary service area
- Major donors
- Medical groups tightly affiliated with the hospital and classified as "senior affiliates"
- Members of the active medical staff, who collectively account for 80 percent of the hospital's admissions
- Full-time employees (designated "associates") who have worked for the organizations more than five years

Employing whatever guidance is provided by the charter, articles of incorporation, precedence, and the organization's own history, your board must identify key stakeholders: those who must be treated as "owners" if the organization is to thrive and whose interests your board is obligated to represent.

We have helped many boards conduct stakeholder analyses. Here are some things we have learned:

- Every conceivable stakeholder shouldn't be specified, just the most important ones.
- The initial process need not be perfect; you can expand and refine selections over time.
- Keep the list short, in most cases under half a dozen.

- Be specific. Describe the characteristics of each stakeholder, and formulate a brief rationale stating why each should be designated an "owner."
- Identify stakeholder groups by the differing interests they have. For example, at first glance, the board of a condominium owners' association might have only one stakeholder: the people who own units in the complex. However, different types of owners (for example, those who reside in their units and those who maintain them as rental properties) have different interests; thus there are in fact several types of stakeholders, not one.
- Recognize that this is hard intellectual work, fraught with tough choices, traps, and blind alleys. Striving for precision regarding who stakeholders are or should be will precipitate some conflict.
- Although stakeholders are typically fairly stable, they can and do change. Your board should therefore periodically review its listing.

The goal is consensus. Your board must agree about the stakeholder groups on whose behalf it governs.

PRINCIPLE 5

The board understands stakeholder interests and expectations.

Once your board has identified stakeholders, it must understand their interests, what they want from and expect of the organization. Specificity is the key; vague generalities are of little value. Your board must be able to answer the following questions:

- To what extent and in what ways is the stakeholder group dependent on the organization? And in what ways is the organization's success dependent on each stakeholder?
- What does each stakeholder expect the organization to accomplish on its behalf?
- How does each stakeholder define organizational success?
- How well does the organization presently meet the expectations and fulfill the needs of each stakeholder? (See Box 3.4.) What specific things must be done to better serve stakeholder interests?

Getting to Great

Box 3.4. Illustrative Stakeholder Interests and Expectations: Sponsoring Religious Community of a Catholic Hospital

- We expect the hospital's clinical programs to conform to the clinical and ethical directives of the Roman Catholic Church.
- We expect the hospital's vision, key goals, and strategies to manifest and personify the guiding principles of the Sisters of St. _____.
- We expect the hospital to achieve an annual net margin from operations of at least x percent.
- We expect that no less than x percent of net profits from operations will be employed to provide care to poor, disadvantaged, and underserved residents in the hospital's primary service area or else made available to the Community Benefit Trust.

We recommend preparing a dossier on each of the key stakeholders, describing them and noting their most important interests and expectations.

PRINCIPLE 6

The board decides and acts on behalf of stakeholders; it discharges its legal fiduciary duty of loyalty.

Identifying stakeholders and understanding their interests is the bedrock of great governance; deliberating and deciding on their behalf, in a manner that furthers their interests, is the most fundamental governance practice.

Statutory and case law holds that boards owe allegiance to stakeholders, acting on their behalf, rather than for personal gain or the benefit of other organizations, groups, or individuals. The dealings of your board must meet two tests. First, it must have good-faith intentions, a desire to serve stakeholders. Second, it must decide in a manner that serves their best interests.

Board members breach their duty of loyalty if, for example, a material conflict of interest influences their decisions, if they seize an opportunity for themselves or other parties that legitimately belongs to the organization, or if they vote to distribute the organization's assets in a way that subverts its purposes, impairs advancing stakeholder interests, or results in private benefit.

Your board can ensure that its duty of loyalty is being discharged in several ways:

- As addressed in Principles 4 and 5, identifying stakeholders and understanding their interests

- Formulating a stakeholder-focused vision and associated goals (see Principles 10 and 11 in Chapter Four)

- Having a policy that defines material conflicts of interest and requires board members to acknowledge such conflicts when they arise (prior to participating in deliberations) and to refrain from discussing, influencing, or voting on matters when such a conflict exits

- Reminding members of their duty of loyalty (and their obligation to act in the best interest of stakeholders) prior to voting on major issues (see Box 3.5)

PRINCIPLE 7

The board discharges its legal fiduciary duty of care.

Not only must your board be loyal to stakeholders, but it must take care in doing so.

The law requires boards to take "due care" in discharging their responsibilities. The board members must be reasonable, diligent, and prudent, and they must demonstrate sound judgment equal to that of ordinary competent persons in similar circumstances. The duty of care focuses on the process of deciding and acting, not the results. The test is to answer the question, Was reasonable care exercised? and not, Were the results optimal, satisfactory, or even tolerable?

Box 3.5. Stakeholder Representatives as Board Members

It is common for health care organizations to include representatives of their most important stakeholder groups as board members. For example, a Catholic health system might designate a specific number of board seats to be filled by members of its sponsoring religious community, or a hospital might designate the chief of staff as an ex officio board member.

This practice can bring a stakeholder perspective into the boardroom and provide valuable knowledge and expertise. However, as discussed more fully in Principle 58 (in Chapter Seven), although such members may come from a particular stakeholder group, they breach their fiduciary duty of loyalty if they serve exclusive as an advocate of that particular stakeholder's interests.

Your board can presume that information, analyses, and recommendations provided by management, staff, and consultants are accurate, truthful, and informed, unless there is compelling reason to believe otherwise.

Courts are very hesitant to substitute their judgment, after the fact, for that of your board. The expectation is simply that board members act carefully, applying common sense and reasonable, informed judgment. Problems typically arise—and these are the areas where the courts' attention is generally focused—regarding matters involving very large expenditures, a fundamental change in mission, acquisitions or mergers, and the disposition of organizational assets.

Here are some ways in which your board can ensure that it is discharging its duty of care:

- Having legal counsel review this fiduciary duty with your board before it begins considering "big deals"
- Making sure that analyses undertaken by staff and consultants thoroughly and accurately portray both the positives and negatives of a proposed initiative

- Distributing background materials well in advance of board meetings so that members can carefully review and reflect on key issues

- Allowing enough time at board meetings for full discussions, questions, elaboration, clarification, deliberation, and debate

- Prior to key votes, conducting an audit of whether your board has exercised its duty of care regarding the matter

PRINCIPLE 8

The board understands the functions it must perform to meet its obligations.

The most important determinant of governance quality is how your board functions. Peter Drucker defines effectiveness as "doing the right things." To be effective, your board must have a precise, coherent, and shared definition of the things it must do to make the most difference (on behalf of stakeholders) and add the greatest value (to the organization).

Governance work has two facets: fulfilling responsibilities and performing roles. *Responsibilities* are the "what" aspects of governance, the substantive issues to which your board must attend. *Roles* are the "how" aspects, the activities your board must perform. Together responsibilities and roles define governance, answering the question, What type of work should my board be doing? (See Figure 3.1.)

Your board has five responsibilities:

- Formulating the organization's *ends,* its vision and key goals, and ensuring that management strategies are aligned with the vision and goals

- Ensuring high levels of *executive performance*

- Ensuring that the organization provides *high-quality care*

- Ensuring the organization's *financial health*

- Ensuring the board's own *effectiveness, efficiency, and creativity* (self)

To fulfill these responsibilities, your board must perform *three roles:*

Figure 3.1. Governance Functions: Board Work

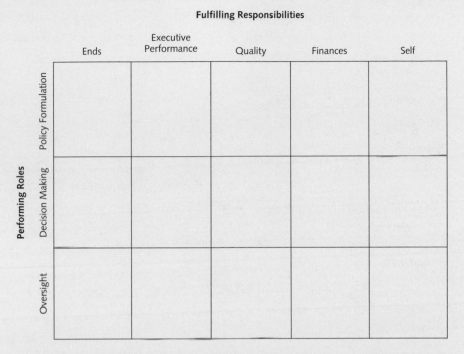

Board work involves three main roles with respect to five primary responsibilities. To meet its obligations to stakeholders, your board must formulate policy for, make decisions about, and oversee the board's ends, executive performance, quality, finances, and effectiveness and efficiency.

- *Policy formulation,* specifying and conveying its expectations and directives
- *Decision making,* choosing among alternatives regarding matters requiring board input
- *Oversight,* monitoring and assessing key organizational process and outcomes

Your board's responsibilities are the focus of Chapter Four; roles will be addressed in Chapter Five.

The types of things your board could do is nearly unlimited; statutory law and court decisions impose few restrictions. However, your board's time and energy are very limited. Thus to focus its attention and leverage its effort, your board must do the type of work that makes the most difference and adds the greatest value—fulfilling its responsibilities and performing its roles.

GOVERNANCE CHECKUP
Obligations

Respond to all items.

	No	Not Entirely	Yes
1. My board understands and fulfills its overarching obligation: representing, advancing, and protecting stakeholder interests.	1	2	3
2. My board has explicitly and precisely identified the organization's key stakeholders.	1	2	3
3. My board understands the expectations and interests of key stakeholders groups.	1	2	3
4. My board discharges its legal fiduciary duty of loyalty; we deliberate, decide, and act on behalf of stakeholders.	1	2	3
5. My board discharges its legal fiduciary duty of care; we act prudently, reasonably, and with informed judgment.	1	2	3
6. Members of my board have a precise, coherent, and shared understanding of the responsibilities we must fulfill and the roles we must perform to meet our obligations.	1	2	3

Total your responses for the six items, divide by 18, and then multiply by 100. The product is your board's percentage of the maximum score in this area.

Total _____ ÷ 18 × 100 = _____ percent

GETTING STARTED

✓ Spend some time at an upcoming meeting discussing your board's fundamental obligation to represent stakeholders and their interests.

What are the practical implications of this obligation?

When and how has your board done this at its best?

What are some instances where this obligation was not met? What were the consequences?

✓ If your board has never conducted a stakeholder analysis or not done so recently, perform one now (see Box 3.6). Start by identifying and understanding the interests and expectations of the organization's most important stakeholders. Such an undertaking, to be done well, will require preparatory staff work. The deliberation itself should probably take place over a half-day at a retreat. Our suggestion is to start small and focus on less than a half-dozen stakeholders.

✓ When major issues and important matters are being discussed, encourage board members to take a stakeholder perspective. Reinforce your board's obligations and its duties of loyalty and care. Board deliberations can become diffused and confused when members argue their individual points of view. Realize that although members must be true to their values, they do not sit on your board to advance their own agendas; their job is to represent stakeholders.

Box 3.6. The Stakeholder Analysis Process

Undertaking an analysis of an organization's stakeholders entails five steps.

Step 1: Consensus Among the Board

Your board must reach consensus that a stakeholder analysis would be beneficial and should be undertaken. Your board must agree that its overarching obligation is to represent the interests of stakeholders, that it cannot govern effectively unless it has identified them and understands their interests, and that governance work must be stakeholder-centric and stakeholder-driven.

Step 2: Specification of Key Stakeholders

The executive committee or an ad hoc committee develops an initial listing of potential stakeholders (we recommend less than half a dozen).

Management prepares a brief description of each stakeholder.

The stakeholder descriptions are distributed to the committee for review and input.

A portion of a board meeting is devoted to discussing and deliberating the initial listing, determining which groups should be included and which should not.

Step 3: Determination of Stakeholder Interests and Expectations

For each of the stakeholders specified, management undertakes an investigation and analysis to identify their most important interests and expectations. This will likely entail interviews with selected stakeholder group representatives, a review of information supplied by such groups (such as annual reports or surveys), and the compilation of publicly available information.

Management then prepares a draft profile for each stakeholder that is reviewed by the committee.

A portion of a board meeting is devoted to discussing the stakeholder profiles and modifying them if necessary.

Step 4: Preparation of Stakeholder Dossiers

A dossier is prepared for each of the stakeholders, including a description, the rationale for identifying them as key stakeholders, and a profile of their most important interests, demands, and expectations. The dossiers are distributed to board members.

Step 5: Discussion of Each Stakeholder

A board meeting is devoted to discussing each stakeholder dossier. Some questions that should be addressed are

- How important is this stakeholder? How dependent is the organization's success on it? Stakeholders are not equal in terms of their power and the demands they can make on the organization.
- How well does the organization presently fulfill the expectations and meet the needs of each stakeholder? In this regard, what are the organization's primary strengths and most pronounced weaknesses? We recommend that the organization be graded from the perspective of each stakeholder.
- What specific things must your board do to better represent each stakeholder? What must the organization do to serve each one better?
- If all stakeholder interests cannot be served in a particular situation, which take precedence and why?

CHAPTER 4

Functioning: Responsibilities

This chapter focuses on half of what your board must do to function effectively: fulfill its responsibilities for ends, executive performance, quality, finances, and its own effectiveness and efficiency(self). The other aspect of functioning, performing roles, is addressed in Chapter Five.

ENDS

PRINCIPLE 9

The board understands the importance of and fulfills its responsibility for determining the organization's ends.

Organizations are means for accomplishing ends. Determining which ends will be pursued and which will not is a board responsibility.

In order to discharge this responsibility, your board must

- Formulate the organization's vision

- Specify its key goals

- Ensure that management strategies will lead to accomplishing key goals and fulfilling the vision

The organization pursues ends on behalf of its stakeholders. Thus if your board has not identified these stakeholders (Principle 4) or does not understand their interests (Principle 5), it cannot formulate meaningful ends on their behalf.

By formulating ends, your board defines the organization, now and in the future. Its other responsibilities (for executive performance, quality, finances, board effectiveness, and efficiency) all flow from this one.

PRINCIPLE 10

The board formulates the organization's vision.

Mention "vision," and what pops into most people's minds is something like this: "We will become a leader in our market, providing the highest-quality care at the lowest possible cost." The concept of vision we will be developing bears no resemblance to this sort of vague and meaningless statement (see Box 4.1).

Although they may differ in a variety of ways, successful organizations have one thing in common: they have precise, coherent, and empowering visions. The reason is simple: an organization cannot achieve what its leaders are unable to envision.

A *vision* is a description of what the organization should become, at its very best. It spells the difference between purposefully moving into the future or aimlessly wandering there. Visions are composed of core purposes and values.

Box 4.1. The Difference Between Vision and Mission

Visions imagine the future, pointing to where an organization *should go*. *Missions* define the present, describing what an organization *is*. Visions challenge; missions anchor. Although both are important, we will focus on vision here. The reason is that the organization cannot alter where it is or has been. Formulating or reformulating the vision is your board's best lever for influencing the organization's future on behalf of its stakeholders.

Core purposes are the most important things your organization wants to achieve. They answer the following questions:

- At its very best, why should the organization exist?

- In what ways should it be different from what it is now? What should it *not* become? How should it remain the same?

- What must the organization do to further the interests of key stakeholders and meet their needs and expectations?

- What types of customers should the organization serve? Whom should it be serving that it is not serving now? What types of customers should be avoided?

- What types of benefits should the organization provide?

Core purposes are not lists of services or objectives (such as market share targets). Rather, they are your organization's reason for being, now and in the future.

Core values are the most important things for which your organization should stand as it goes about achieving its purpose. To determine your core values, answer the following questions:

- At our very best, what principles should guide the organization's decisions and actions?

- How should the organization behave (and not behave) in its relationships with stakeholders, regulators, customers, purchasers, partners, competitors, the medical staff, and employees?

- What are the ultimate "thou shalts" and "thou shalt nots" the organization should respect?

- What values should define the organization's heart and soul? What rules should it live by?

An empowering and useful vision is

- *Specific, precise, and detailed*—a fine-grained picture, not an abstract painting, of what the organization should look like

- *Self-actualizing*—a description of the organization at its very best
- *Future-oriented*—focusing on the future, not the present or the past

Your board must craft the organization's vision (see Box 4.2). Management *should not* do the "heavy lifting," drafting a statement that is briefly

---

Box 4.2. Elements of a Vision: Purposes and Values

Here are some core purposes and values for a Catholic short-term hospital.

Core Purposes

- Providing the poor, uninsured, and underinsured in our community with health promotion, preventive, and curative services equal in quality and comprehensiveness to those provided to individuals with standard insurance coverage, at no out-of-pocket cost
- Offering, in cooperation with our partners, an array of health care services perceived by payers and purchasers in the top quartile in terms of value
- Being viewed as the employer of choice in our community; providing employees opportunities for meaningful work and continual development at rates of compensation that exceed the norm for comparable positions
- Funding community organizations, agencies, and programs that prevent disease, promote health, and enhance wellness

Core Values

- Respecting the dignity and worth of all people
- Being honest and fair in our dealings with everyone
- Creating collaborative and mutually empowering relationships with employees and members of our medical staff
- Infusing the compassion and caring of Christ into every aspect of the curing and caring process
- Treating competitors the same way we would want to be treated by them
- Being viewed by our community as an exemplary corporate citizen

---

reviewed and then approved by your board after superficial discussion and deliberation. Your board must be proactive and engaged in developing its vision of the organization on behalf of stakeholders.

Yet this is not an area where your board can go it alone. The formulation of a great vision depends on careful and thorough analyses of the organization's strengths, weaknesses, opportunities, and threats, both internal and external. Management lays the groundwork for your board's visioning by doing the necessary preparatory "staff work."

Generating a vision is often inhibited by the attempt to produce an elegant statement. The emphasis becomes wordsmithing rather than substance. Accordingly, we recommend beginning by drafting bulleted lists of what your organization's purposes and values should be, initially not exceeding a half-dozen items each. Don't try for perfection! Attempting to craft the perfect vision statement will stall and then undermine your producing a usable one. Get started; do something. Regard everything you write as a work in progress that will be continually elaborated on and refined over time.

PRINCIPLE 11

The board specifies key organizational goals.

Visioning will amount to little in the absence of clearly and precisely specified key goals. *Goals* are "specific accomplishables," the most important things the organization must achieve to fulfill its vision. Your board's formulation of key goals increases the richness and density of its vision, saying to management and the medical staff, "Above all else, accomplish these things."

Key organizational goals should be

- *Few in number*—in most instances less than a dozen; focusing on only the most vision-critical things your board wants accomplished

- *Realistically achievable*—but stretching the organization's capacities, competencies, and potential

- *Quantifiable*—providing precise targets and clear measures of success or the lack thereof

- *Time-specific*—noting when they should be achieved; most board-formulated key goals need not be annual, as truly important ones can take years to accomplish

- *Consistent*—so that accomplishing one goal does not impair achieving others

- *Brief, crisply worded, and unequivocal*—so that there can be no confusion about what is expected

- *Reviewed and, if necessary, modified annually*—despite their relatively long "shelf life"; if the situation and organizational challenges change, so should goals

Your board has an obligation to formulate and articulate the most important things it expects the organization to accomplish (see Box 4.3). In

---

Box 4.3. Sample Organizational Goals for a Short-Term Hospital

- To remain a freestanding enterprise not merged with or acquired by a larger integrated health care delivery system.
- To have 250 physicians in our owned or tightly affiliated medical groups by the end of 2005.
- To complete implementation of a patient safety system by January 2004.
- To consummate the sale or disposition of our wholly owned HMO under the most favorable terms possible by December 2003.
- To achieve a AA+ bond rating by June 2003.
- To be rated in the top 10 percent of our peer group on the (standardized quality report), the (standardized patient satisfaction report), the (standardized employee satisfaction report), and the (standardized medical staff satisfaction report) by the end of 2005.

---

addition, strategies (to which we turn next) cannot be developed unless key goals have been specified.

PRINCIPLE 12

The board does not become involved in developing organizational strategies; this task is delegated to management.

Ask a board member (or an executive for that matter) whether a board should be involved in strategy, and the answer you generally get is "Of course!" Boards must be strategically minded and focused, but they should *not* be directly involved in the development of specific strategies.

Strategies are plans for allocating the organization's resources to accomplish goals.

Just as formulation of a vision and the specification of goals are the board's responsibilities, developing strategy is management's. It demands time and technical expertise in addition to knowledge about the market, customers, patients, competitors, and the organization's own capacities that exceeds those possessed by even the very best boards.

Should your board then wash its hands of all things strategic? Certainly not. Here are our recommendations:

- Each year, management develops a set of core organizational strategies. The individual strategies should be accompanied by a concise rationale stating how each is linked to accomplishing one or more board-formulated goals and fulfilling the vision.

- Core strategies (and accompanying rationales) are then reviewed by your board. The questions it must address are these: Is each strategy aligned with key goals and the vision and likely to achieve them? Is the rationale sound? If for any reason the answer is no, the strategy is sent back to management for modification.

This approach—having your board focus on vision and goals and having management develop strategy—effectively subdivides and coordinates

Box 4.4. Governance and Management Work

Governance and management are fundamentally different but complementary organizational functions. Here is the distinction: the board appreciates the difference between running an organization and seeing that it is well run. Management is the former, governance is the latter.

The single most important decision your board makes (over and over again) is where to draw the line between governance and management work. If the bar is set too high, your board abdicates its responsibility. If the bar is positioned too low, your board becomes overwhelmed by taking on tasks it is unable to perform well.

The principles dealing with your board's obligations and responsibility for ends illustrate this key point. To optimize its effectiveness and leverage, your board should focus its limited attention, time, and energy on identifying stakeholders and understanding their interests, formulating a vision, and specifying key goals. Boards have the collective perspective, competency, and wisdom to do these things. And doing them adds real value to the organization on behalf of its stakeholders. Management should then focus on developing strategy. It has the time, expertise, and knowledge to do so, whereas the board does not.

---

governance and management responsibilities, eliminates duplication of effort, and minimizes conflict (see Box 4.4).

CHECKUP
Ends
Respond to all items.

	No	Not Entirely	Yes
1. My board appreciates the importance and nature of its responsibility for ends.	1	2	3

2. My board has formulated a detailed, 1   2   3
   precise, and empowering vision for the
   organization, specifying its core purposes
   and values.

3. My board has specified key 1   2   3
   organizational goals that
   must be accomplished to fulfill
   the vision.

4. My board does not develop strategies; 1   2   3
   rather, it assesses the extent to which
   management strategies are aligned with
   key goals and the vision and likely to
   achieve them.

Total your responses for the four items, divide by 12, and then multiply by 100. The product is your board's percentage of the maximum score in this area.

Total _____ ÷ 12 × 100 = _____ percent

GETTING STARTED

✔ Devote time at an upcoming board meeting and assess your organization's vision and key goals. Answer the following questions:

How long has it been since the they were seriously reworked?

Has your board been involved in formulating them, or has this task been delegated (either by design or default) to management?

Are the vision and goals an expression of stakeholder interests?

Does the vision crisply and clearly state core purposes and values? Is it a rich description of what your organization should "look like," at its very best, in the future?

Are goals truly key, the organization's most vision-critical accomplishables? Are they few in number, achievable, quantifiable, time-specific, consistent, and brief?

✓ If your organization's vision and key goals don't "pass muster," consider holding a half-day board retreat to brainstorm an initial list of core purposes, core values, and key goals. They can be reworked and embellished by an ad hoc committee and then presented to the full board for discussion, input, and adoption.

EXECUTIVE PERFORMANCE

PRINCIPLE 13

The board understands the importance of and fulfills its responsibility for ensuring high levels of executive performance.

Your board's job is governing, not managing. Indeed, the more it manages, the less it will govern; eventual losers are the organization and its stakeholders.

Yet your board is responsible and accountable for ensuring that the organization is well managed. In order to fulfill this responsibility, your board must

- Recruit and select the chief executive officer (CEO)
- Specify its performance expectations of the CEO
- Assess the CEO's performance
- Periodically adjust the CEO's compensation
- Be prepared, should the need arise, to terminate the CEO's employment relationship with the organization

In fulfilling this responsibility, the objective of your board should be to create a context in which the CEO can maximize his or her performance and contributions, develop a relationship such that your board empowers the CEO and the CEO empowers your board, and focus the CEO's attention and energy on fulfilling the vision and accomplishing key goals on behalf of stakeholders.

PRINCIPLE 14

The CEO is the board's only direct report.

Your board should have only one direct report, the CEO; all other employees are accountable, directly or indirectly, to the CEO. This creates a clear chain of command that minimizes mixed signals and conflict.

Certain implications flow from this principle:

- Your board, and individual board members, should neither make requests of nor direct other management staff.

- The recruitment and selection of management team members should be the responsibility of the CEO or of people who report to the CEO.

- Your board should not become directly involved in assessing the performance or adjusting the compensation of other management staff.

This principle once again underscores the importance of your board's drawing a clear distinction between governance and management work (recall Box 4.4).

PRINCIPLE 15

When a vacancy occurs, the board selects the CEO.

When the position becomes vacant, recruiting and selecting a CEO is one of the most important tasks your board will ever undertake. This decision has a singularly significant impact on your board's success and that of the organization. Top performers are hard to find, and the best people are generally not seeking new positions. Until a new CEO is in place, the organization's operational metabolism slows down, and key strategic issues are typically put on hold. Most board members who have been involved in a CEO search report that it is one of the most time-consuming, stressful, and challenging aspects of governance work.

The search process requires special expertise, contacts, experience, perspectives, and time that boards typically do not possess. Therefore, we strongly recommend retaining a search consultant to assist with the process.

We have observed and participated in a number of executive searches. Here are a few guidelines for a successful search:

- Appoint an ad hoc search committee composed only of board members; the executive committee could take on this task. The search committee should be led by the board chairperson.

- Reserve decision making to the board. Although the search committee can do much of the preparatory work, selecting finalist candidates and extending an offer are decisions that should be made by the board.

- Base your recruitment, screening, and selection on a precise and explicit specification of the competencies and capacities needed to lead the organization into its future, fulfilling its vision and accomplishing key goals; the extent to which a candidate's values mesh with those of the organization; and professional and personal characteristics and experience deemed critical by the board.

- Look for winners. The single best predictor of future success is past success, so pay attention to the track records of candidates. Have they led other organizations down the path that yours wants to travel?

PRINCIPLE 16

The board has a CEO succession plan.

CEO departure (due to death, retirement, resignation, or removal) is something that most boards do not like to think about or plan for. Often the response is "We'll cross that bridge when we come to it." Vacancies in the top slot usually arise unexpectedly and seem to occur at the worst possible moment; surprised reaction to this, rather than thoughtful advanced planning, is costly and disruptive to the organization.

"Be prepared" is excellent advice. Your board should have a CEO succession plan that specifies all of the following:

- The management team member who will assume the CEO's duties on an interim basis

- How the present responsibilities of the interim CEO appointee will be distributed to other members of the management team (failure is assured when someone attempts to hold down several jobs simultaneously)

- If and how the interim CEO's compensation will be temporarily adjusted to reflect additional responsibilities

44

- If the CEO held a board seat, whether the interim CEO will assume it
- Whether the interim CEO should be encouraged to apply for the permanent position or discouraged or even prohibited from doing so

Your board CEO succession plan should be reviewed every several years.

PRINCIPLE 17

The board specifies its key expectations of the CEO.

As its only direct report, the CEO is accountable to your board for carrying out its policies and decisions. Accordingly, your board must explicitly and precisely convey what it expects of and wants from the CEO. We are continually amazed at how few boards engage in this absolutely essential governance practice. Illustrative expectations are presented in Box 4.5.

Here are some guidelines:

- Specify only the most important expectations, those that must be met by the CEO to do a great job in the eyes of your board and on behalf of stakeholders.
- Craft expectations that are operational and incorporate quantitative benchmarks, if possible. But do not avoid specifying subjective expectations just because they can't be precisely measured.
- Focus on things over which the CEO has control.
- Involve the CEO in the process.
- Update and revise your board's expectations annually.
- Codify your expectations. Reducing them to writing encourages precision and provides a vehicle for conveying to the CEO what your board deems most important.

PRINCIPLE 18

Employing explicit criteria, the board assesses the CEO's performance and contributions annually.

Box 4.5. Board Expectations of the CEO: A Sample

- The CEO is prohibited from engaging in or knowingly allowing management staff or employees to engage in any act that is unethical, illegal, or in violation of board policy.
- The CEO is expected to keep the board informed of all important matters affecting the organization's vision-critical strategic, financial, operational, and clinical performance and to deal with the board under the doctrine of "no surprises."
- The CEO is expected to be involved in the community as demonstrated by serving in a leadership capacity in at least two community-focused organizations.
- The CEO is expected to behave in all professional and personal dealings in a way that brings credit to the organization.
- The CEO is expected to participate in at least thirty hours of formal continuing professional education each year.
- The CEO is expected to groom one member of the management team who could, if the need arose, assume the CEO position on an interim basis.
- The CEO and members of his or her immediate family are prohibited from accepting any gifts, gratuities, or other considerations that have a value exceeding $100 from parties doing or seeking to do business with the organization.

Board members continually evaluate the CEO's performance; that's unavoidable. The problem is that such assessments are often sporadic, idiosyncratic, and focused on isolated events and behaviors.

Designing and employing a formal, regular CEO performance assessment process is essential, as it gives your board its best opportunity for better understanding the CEO's responsibilities and challenges; focusing the CEO's attention and energy on what really matters; clarifying mutual expectations; providing the CEO with feedback, direction, and affirmation; encouraging continuing professional development; and constructing the basis for adjustment of the CEO's compensation.

Your board cannot undertake a meaningful assessment of the CEO's performance unless the necessary prerequisites are in place: a fully fleshed out vision, clear and measurable organizational goals, precise strategies, and specific CEO performance expectations. The process must be designed to help your board answer two questions:

- Over the past year, to what extent has the CEO contributed to the organization's vision being fulfilled (Principle 10), key goals being accomplished (Principle 11), strategies being pursued (Principle 12), and financial objectives being achieved (Principle 28)?

- To what extent did the CEO meet the board's performance expectations (Principle 17)?

We suggest the following:

- In line with Principle 14, your board should assess only the CEO's performance.

- A committee may do the groundwork, but your board should thoroughly discuss and approve the completed evaluation.

- The CEO should be a partner in the process, not an object of it. He or she should have a voice (although not the final say) in developing performance assessment criteria.

- The CEO should undertake an assessment of his or her own performance, which should then be used by your board as one input in formulating its evaluation.

- Your board must provide the CEO with explicit and candid feedback and work with the CEO to develop an action plan to improve performance and contributions.

PRINCIPLE 19

The board adjusts the CEO's compensation annually.

Appraisal of the CEO's performance provides the basis for adjusting his or her compensation. Technique, method, tax considerations, and legalities can be overwhelming. Accordingly, this is an area where it is easy to lose sight of what is most important.

To be effective, your board's approach to compensation must be based on a clearly articulated philosophy that answers the following questions:

- How is the CEO's compensation intended to further stakeholder interests and facilitate accomplishing the organization's vision, goals, strategies, and financial objectives?

- At what level, relative to executives in similar organizations, should the CEO's base salary be set? That is, as a general rule, does your board want to pay above, at, or below the market?

- What proportion of total compensation should be based on performance, and what criteria should be employed to determine the amount of incentive compensation?

- What types and amounts of fringe benefits are provided?

- What are the terms and conditions of the CEO's severance package?

Here's what we recommend:

- CEO compensation should be viewed as an important investment in the organization's future, not an expense. Value added to the organization by the CEO should be a huge multiple of his or her total compensation. Your board must be prudent, but it should not be "penny wise and pound foolish."

- Your board must have a clear rationale for the amount of CEO compensation provided and how it was determined. Internal Revenue Service guidelines for nonprofit organizations prohibit compensation arrangements that amount to private inurement or the distribution of excess revenue that should benefit stakeholders. Compensation judged to be "unreasonable" or "unjustified" can result in civil penalties and may jeopardize the organization's tax-exempt status.

- Specific terms of the compensation arrangement should be codified in a written employment contract.

PRINCIPLE 20

Should the need arise, the board is willing and able to terminate the CEO's employment with the organization.

A CEO's employment can be ended for four reasons: death or disability, retirement, leaving to take another position, or forced termination. A board ordinarily accepts the first three (typically with regret), but it must initiate the last.

Your board must have confidence in and support the CEO. When this is no longer possible and the situation is irreversible, the CEO must be removed without delay. Stringing out the process deflects the attention of your board, causes unnecessary conflict, impairs the functioning of other managers and staff, slows down the organization, and is unfair to the CEO.

Termination should be "for cause," of which there are three justifiable grounds:

- Disregard for your board's responsibility and authority as demonstrated by the CEO's repeatedly and consciously violating the board's policies and directives

- A pattern of inability to meet your board's performance expectations and facilitate fulfilling the vision, accomplishing goals, pursuing key strategies, and achieving financial objectives

- Unethical or illegal behavior

Except in the event of illegal or unethical behavior, a decision to terminate the CEO should rarely be made on the basis of a single incident or outcome.

Termination should always be handled with dignity and respect, recognizing the CEO's past efforts and accomplishments.

CHECKUP

Executive Performance

Respond to all items.

	No	Not Entirely	Yes
1. My board understands the nature and importance of its responsibility for ensuring high levels of executive performance.	1	2	3
2. The CEO is the only employee who is directly accountable to my board.	1	2	3
3. My board would be able to undertake an effective CEO recruitment and selection process if the need arose.	1	2	3
4. My board has a CEO succession plan in place.	1	2	3
5. My board has specified its key performance expectations of the CEO.	1	2	3
6. Employing specific criteria, my board annually assesses the CEO's performance and provides explicit feedback and coaching.	1	2	3
7. My board employs a formal process to adjust the CEO's compensation annually.	1	2	3
8. Should the need arise, my board would be prepared to terminate the CEO's employment relationship.	1	2	3

Total your responses for the eight items, divide by 24, and then multiply by 100. The product is your board's percentage of the maximum score in this area.

Total _____ ÷ 24 × 100 = _____ percent

GETTING STARTED

✓ Consider having your board meet in executive session, without the CEO present, several times a year. Schedule this so it is a planned periodic event and is recognized as such by the CEO. This is your board's opportunity to talk candidly about the CEO's performance (both positives and negatives) and what should be done to continually enhance it. The chair should then provide the CEO with feedback and recommendations.

✓ If your board does not have a CEO succession plan, formulate one.

✓ Craft an initial set of CEO performance expectations. Identify the most important things the CEO must do and accomplish in order to be judged successful by your board.

✓ Consider retaining a consultant to work with your board in designing and implementing an effective CEO compensation system. There is an added benefit here: the CEO can leverage the consultant's work to design or redesign the assessment and compensation of other executives and key staff.

✓ If your board does not have an employment contract with the CEO, develop one.

✓ Arrange a time in a relaxed setting where your board can have a candid conversation with the CEO about the strengths and weaknesses of the board-CEO relationship and what should be done to enhance it (see Box 4.6).

QUALITY

PRINCIPLE 21

The board understands that it is ultimately responsible for ensuring the quality of patient care provided in and by the organization.

Responsibility for ensuring quality is unique to the boards of organizations that provide health care services. Other nonprofit organizations and com-

Box 4.6. Nature and Strength of the Board-CEO Relationship

- Does the CEO appreciate the importance of governance and the contribution your board can make to his or her own success and that of the organization?
- To what extent is the CEO knowledgeable about governance functioning, structure, composition, and infrastructure?
- To what extent does the CEO (in collaboration with the chair) exercise governance leadership, stimulating and facilitating high levels of board performance and contributions?
- What are the CEO's greatest strengths in working with your board?
- To what extent does your board trust the CEO? Trust can be defined as the experience of seeing commitments fulfilled. Is the CEO credible and honest in his or her dealings with your board?
- What are the CEO's most pronounced weaknesses in working with your board?
- Does the CEO provide the right amounts and types of information to your board so that it can fulfill its responsibilities? What should the CEO be doing differently or better in this area?
- What things should the CEO be doing to create a better board and more capable board members?
- Does an effective functional partnership exist between your board and the CEO? That is, are your board and the CEO mutually supportive and empowering?

mercial corporation boards can delegate this to management. Because of the presence of a voluntary medical staff (who in most instances are not employees) and due to legislative mandates, court decisions, regulations, and accreditation standards, health care organization boards bear the ultimate responsibility for quality.

This aspect of governance typically causes board members their greatest concern because of the complexity and mystique of medical work, and most board members, lacking clinical expertise, find it unreasonable to be asked to pass judgment on the competency, experience, performance, and outcomes of individual physicians.

To fulfill this responsibility, your board must

- Have a precise and shared working definition of quality
- Credential members of the medical staff
- Ensure that quality monitoring and management systems are in place and functioning effectively
- Employ specific quantitative indicators and standards to assess the quality of care provided and when problems are detected, make sure that corrective action is undertaken
- Ensure that a plan is in place to continually improve quality

Your board must be able to answer three questions: What is quality? Does your organization provide it? How do you know?

PRINCIPLE 22

The board has developed a precise and explicit working definition of quality.

Quality is an illusive concept, difficult to pin down (see Box 4.7). It means different things to different people. However, if your board fails to define quality, it will be unable to measure it; and things that are not measured cannot be continuously improved.

Thus the challenge is to develop an explicit and precise working definition of quality that provides the foundation for quantifying, measuring, continuously improving, and ultimately ensuring it.

Quality has different dimensions; here are just a few:

- *Focus*—individuals versus populations or communities
- *Aspect*—the process of providing care versus the outcomes of that care
- *Component*—medical content versus the experience of receiving it
- *Orientation*—promoting and maintaining health versus curing disease

Box 4.7. What Is Quality Anyway? Two Perspectives

At a recent meeting, the board received two reports regarding the quality of a rapidly expanding off-site outpatient surgery program.

The first was from the medical staff chief, who reported on the results of a detailed six-month study that conclusively demonstrated that quality, as measured by thirty-five widely used and valid clinical benchmarks, was superb. The program ranked in the 95th percentile overall when compared with its peer group.

The second report, from the hospital's director of marketing, presented data indicating that the program generated more patient complaints than any other area in the past year. She shared a study commissioned to help staff identify the problem and understand it better. The study was conducted by a reputable consulting firm doing patient satisfaction analysis, using a questionnaire validated over the course of five years with hundreds of clients. It showed that patients perceived the program's quality in the lowest quartile on a host of measures, including scheduling convenience, waiting time prior to service, interaction with staff, nurse attentiveness, and clarity of physician instructions regarding medications and aftercare.

In addition, overall quality and aspects of it can be perceived differently by various stakeholders, customers, and purchasers, such as patients, families, physicians, nurses, employees, insurers and health plans, accrediting bodies, regulators, and buyers.

These different perceptions of quality should be viewed as an opportunity rather than a problem. They provide the means for your board to develop a working definition of quality that is most relevant to your organization. The process is one of triangulation; of getting a navigational fix by comparing measurements taken from different directions simultaneously. Developing a meaningful definition of quality entails

- Identifying key stakeholders and customers
- Understanding what they want and expect from the organization in terms of the different aspects of care
- Prioritizing and balancing these specifications
- Shaping them into your board's working definition of quality
- Periodically redefining quality as needs and expectations change

Employing this process, the elusive concept of quality is defined practically, specifically, and comprehensively. The resulting definition grounds and focuses your board's attention. It provides the necessary foundation and framework for credentialing physicians, ensuring that necessary quality systems and plans are in place, and assessing the quality of care provided.

PRINCIPLE 23

Based on recommendations of the medical staff and after a careful, thorough, and independent review, the board credentials physicians.

This is a complex process that due to the constraints of space will receive only a small measure of the attention it warrants. We refer you to two resources on the topic in Box 4.8.

Box 4.8. Credentialing Resources

- *The Board's Role in Quality of Care: A Practical Guide for Hospital Trustees,* by James E. Orlikoff and Mary K. Totten (Chicago: American Hospital Publishing, 1991)

- *Quality from the Top: Working with Hospital Governing Boards to Assure Quality,* by James E. Orlikoff (Chicago: Pluribus Press, 1990)

Credentialing is the process that leads to the initial appointment, reappointment, and privilege delineation of physicians (and in some cases, other categories of licensed practitioners). It requires the coordinated activities and actions of many groups in the organization, including the individual practitioner, the medical staff office, the quality and utilization management department, the clinical division in which the practitioner is or will be working, the medical staff executive or credentials committee, the board quality committee, and your board. The key aspects of this process, which vary from institution to institution, are depicted in Figure 4.1.

The objective of this process is to assist your board in making two decisions: *which* physicians will be appointed or reappointed to the organiza-

Figure 4.1. The Credentialing Process

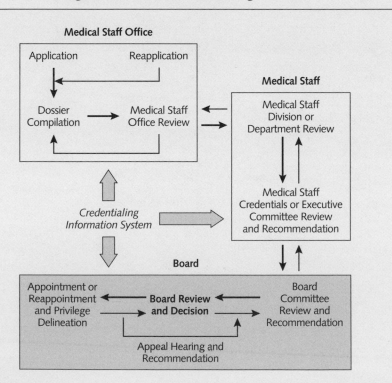

tion's medical staff and allowed to admit and treat patients (eligibility to practice) and *what* they will be allowed to do (scope of competent practice).

The parameters of effective credentialing have been established over the past thirty years through a series of court decisions, regulations, and accrediting criteria. Reduced to the basics, they are as follows:

- Your board must make final appointment, reappointment, and privilege delineation decisions. All steps of the process prior to the board's action are supportive and advisory, designed to gather and analyze data and make recommendations.

- Board credentialing decisions must be made on a case-by-case basis after a thorough, careful, and independent review. This detailed review can be conducted by a board committee, but the final action must be taken by your board as a whole.

- Your board is accountable for ensuring the effectiveness and fairness of the entire credentialing process, not just the steps in which it is directly involved.

You might be thinking, I'm not a clinician, so how, as a board member, can I possibly make intelligent decisions about who's a good physician and who's not? The answer lies in the proper distribution of credentialing tasks between your board and the medical staff. Simply stated, the medical staff gathers data, conducts analyses, and prepares recommendations; your board, typically aided by a committee, verifies that the medical staff has done its job right and makes the final decisions.

The medical staff's role is to receive applications or reapplications and to collect needed information on them. Employing specific criteria, each practitioner's qualifications, experience, performance, and outcomes are assessed. The staff then forwards a recommendation, along with a summary analysis, to your board.

Your board's role is to ensure that a fair and effective credentialing process and criteria are in place. It compares results of the criteria-based review with the medical staff's recommendation regarding each applicant. When all indications are consistent, your board approves the recommendation. When they appear to be inconsistent, your board requests additional information and analyses, sends the application back to the medical staff for further review, or rejects the recommendation.

PRINCIPLE 24

The board makes sure that necessary quality and utilization management systems are in place and functioning effectively.

The objective of a quality management system is to monitor, assess, and improve the process of providing care and its outcomes. It should answer three questions:

- Do the clinical practices, processes, and outcomes meet or exceed current professional standards?

- What initiatives should be undertaken to correct any deficiencies and improve quality?

- What were the results of these initiatives?

A utilization management system monitors, assesses, and ensures the efficient use of resources employed in providing care. It focuses on such things as the necessity and timing of admission decisions, length of stay, level of care, services provided and procedures performed, appropriateness and timing of discharge, and nature of follow-up care.

Your board should review the adequacy of these systems yearly. The questions addressed might include these:

- What quality and utilization goals or objectives have been developed? How well aligned are they with your board's definition of quality in addition to its vision and key goals?

- Are resources (personnel, equipment and systems) adequate for achieving the stated goals and objectives?

- What major activities (reviews, studies, audits) will be undertaken over the next year, and what are they intended to accomplish?

- What measuring, monitoring, assessment, and management systems are in place? Are they adequate? What changes are needed?

• How are quality and utilization systems integrated and coordinated?

PRINCIPLE 25

Employing specific and quantitative indicators and standards, the board assesses the quality of care and, if problems are detected, demands corrective action.

Defining quality, credentialing members of the medical staff, and ensuring the effectiveness of quality and utilization management systems culminate in your board's direct involvement in assessing the quality of care. It is a four-step process:

• *Step 1.* Based on work performed by and input from management and the medical staff, your board develops a panel of quality indicators. Health care organizations collect extensive amounts of quality data. Your board's challenge is to select indicators (see Box 4.9) that are representative, comprehensive, quantifiable, valid, and most important, aligned with its definition of quality.

• *Step 2.* For each indicator, a standard is specified: a level that the indicator should achieve, not exceed or fall below. Standards can be obtained from a variety of sources, including published national norms (from federal and state agencies, commercial vendors, and accrediting groups), peer group comparisons, or the organization's own past performance.

• *Step 3.* Trends in variations between indicators and standard are compared and analyzed.

• *Step 4.* If problems are detected, your board requires that management or the medical staff (or both) develop plans to correct them.

Broader aspects of quality monitoring and assessment process are addressed in Chapter Five (Principle 37, dealing with your board's oversight role).

Box 4.9. Quality Indicators

Quality indicators must be tailored to the organization and grounded on your board's definition of quality. Here are some examples of quality indicators:

- Hospital acquired infection rate
- Medication error rate
- Severity-adjusted mortality rate by selected procedures
- Percentage of newborns weighing less than 2.5 kilograms
- Average urgent care center waiting time (from check-in to point of first contact with a clinician)
- Average patient, employee, and medical staff satisfaction rate (as measured by an appropriate questionnaire)
- Likelihood that a discharged patient would use the hospital again
- Nurse turnover rate, by personnel category (RN, LPN) and unit
- Nursing position vacancy rate
- Number of nursing registry hours used as a proportion of total full-time nurse hours worked
- Severity-adjusted cost per discharge for each disease category (when combined) accounting for 80 percent of the hospital's volume
- Proportion of individuals in the hospital's primary service area who engage in some form of strenuous exercise at least two times per week
- Unmarried teen pregnancy rate in the hospital's primary service area

PRINCIPLE 26

The board ensures that the organization has a plan for improving quality.

Your board is ultimately responsible not only for the quality of care per se but also for the organization's ongoing effort to continuously improve it. To succeed, the organization must have strategic, operational, and financial plans. These are developed by management and are periodically reviewed by your board. This must also be the case with quality. Accordingly, we recommend that an annual plan for improving quality be submitted to and reviewed by your board. The different approaches that can be employed are described in Box 4.10.

Box 4.10. Types of Quality Improvement Plans

Quality enhancement plans can employ two different approaches.

The *problem-focused approach* is based on inspection and entails a four-step process:

1. Identifying quality problems after they have occurred
2. Investigating and assessing each problem's magnitude, scope, consequences, and cause
3. Undertaking initiatives to correct the problem by making changes in systems, procedures, and practices
4. Monitoring the results and taking follow-up actions as necessary

The *continuous total approach*—also referred to as total quality management (TQM) or continuous quality improvement (CQI)—holds that quality cannot be "inspected in" after the fact; rather, it must be built in throughout the process. It has four key aspects:

1. Understanding the nature of desired outcomes from the customer's perspective
2. Identifying, measuring, and analyzing variations in outcomes
3. Studying the care process (typically with the assistance of employee teams) to isolate the causes of variations
4. Designing sustained initiatives to continuously improve the process so that variations are reduced and outcomes are improved

The quality plans of most health care organizations typically incorporate both approaches.

CHECKUP
Quality

	No	Not Entirely	Yes
1. My board understands the importance and nature of its responsibility for ensuring the quality of care provided in and by the organization	1	2	3
2. My board has formulated a working definition of quality that incorporates the perspectives of customers, purchasers, and clinical professionals.	1	2	3
3. My board bases final decisions regarding the appointment, reappointment, and privileges of physicians on an explicit process, precise criteria, and medical staff recommendations.	1	2	3
4. My board periodically reviews the organization's quality and utilization monitoring and management systems.	1	2	3
5. My board has a specified set of measurable quality indicators and standards and employs them to assess the quality of care provided in and by the organization.	1	2	3
6. My board reviews the organization's plans for improving quality every year.	1	2	3

Total your responses for the six items, divide by 18, and then multiply by 100. The product is your board's percentage of the maximum score in this area.

Total _____ $\div 18 \times 100 =$ _____ percent

GETTING STARTED

✓ Conduct a discussion regarding how, and how well, your board is discharging its responsibility for ensuring quality.

How much has your board been concerned with quality in the past?

How is attending to quality linked with your board's obligation to stakeholders and its responsibility for formulating organizational ends and ensuring financial health?

What is the quality of care provided in and by your organization? Has it been increasing or decreasing over time? How do you know?

On what basis does your board make judgments about quality?

✓ Taking into consideration the perspectives of various key stakeholders and customer groups in addition to the different aspects of quality, develop a rough working definition of quality for the organization. Formulate this definition as a list of specific attributes.

✓ Conduct an audit of the organization's credentialing process. You can do this either by employing internal resources or by retaining a consultant; we recommend doing the latter at least every five years. Have the auditor submit the following information to your board:

A thorough description and mapping of the total credentialing process; we find that many board members do not understand the process and consequently have little confidence in it

A description and an assessment of the specific criteria employed by the medical staff (divisions or departments, credentials or executive committees) to frame their appointment, reappointment, and privilege delineation recommendations

An assessment of the analysis or review undertaken by your board's quality committee

A list of the strengths and weaknesses of the entire process

Recommendations for improving the process

✔ Develop an initial set of no more than a dozen key indicators and associated standards your board can begin employing to measure, monitor, and assess quality.

✔ Ask management to talk with your board about its plans for continually improving quality and the systems that are in place to do so.

FINANCES

PRINCIPLE 27

The board understands the importance of and fulfills its responsibility for ensuring the organization's financial health.

Money is both a health care organization's source of buoyancy and its propellant. Your board must make sure that there is enough and that it is allocated in effective and legitimate ways; your board is accountable to stakeholders for ensuring the organization's financial health. In order to fulfill this responsibility, your board must

- Specify key financial objectives
- Ensure that management-developed budgets will accomplish financial objectives
- Assess the organization's financial performance and outcomes
- Ensure that necessary financial controls are in place and functioning effectively

PRINCIPLE 28

The board specifies key financial objectives for the organization.

Responsibility for "the money" begins with answering three questions: What is your board's definition of financial health? What must the organization accomplish financially to fulfill its vision and accomplish key goals? How should financial performance be assessed?

Each year, your board, typically assisted by its finance committee and with input and counsel from the CEO and chief financial officer, should formulate a set of financial objectives for the organization. They should be comprehensive, covering all areas of financial performance and outcomes; precise and explicit, stating what your board expects; specifically linked to the vision and key goals; and quantifiable, so that the extent to which they have been accomplished can be measured.

Objectives should be developed in four areas:

- *Bottom line*—quarterly and year-end total, operating and nonoperating margins for the organization as a whole, in addition to major lines of business or organizational components

- *Cash*—the amount of cash that should be available by quarter and at year's end

- *Capital*—relative priority that should be given to major investments in facilities and equipment

- *Performance*—targets for an array of ratios (calculated from the balance sheet, income and expense statement, and operating statistics) that measure specific aspects of the organization's financial health

Illustrations of financial objectives are provided in Box 4.11.

Precise financial objectives convey what your board expects and provide management with the framework and guidelines it needs to develop financial plans.

PRINCIPLE 29

The board ensures that management-devised budgets are aligned with financial objectives and the organization's key goals and vision.

Budgets are plans for allocating organizational resources to achieve financial objectives. As with the formulation of strategy (Principle 12), boards should not become directly involved in developing budgets; this is most effectively and efficiently performed by management.

Box 4.11. Sample Financial Objectives

- The organization will achieve an overall net profit from operations of at least x percent.
- Operating revenues will grow at a rate of not less than x percent per year.
- A third-generation cost accounting system will be installed by the third quarter of 2002.
- The organization will achieve a return on equity of not less than x percent.
- Total earnings before interest, taxes, depreciation, and amortization from all for-profit subsidiaries will increase by at least x percent per year over the next five years.
- Severity-adjusted cost per inpatient discharge will be reduced by x percent over the next three years.
- Net yield on investment income (adjusted for inflation, less transaction and management fees) will be at least x percent.

Management's financial planning culminates in the preparation of annual operating, cash, and capital budgets. Boards are typically required to review and approve them. Overwhelmed by their weight, detail, and complexity and the amount of effort that went into preparing them, boards often approach this task as more symbolic than substantive. How, then, does your board exercise appropriate influence on behalf of stakeholders in this process? Here are some suggestions:

- The types of financial information and budgets that management needs to run the organization are very different from those your board requires to govern it. Management, with direction and input from the board's finance committee, should prepare a "governance-friendly" and focused budget for your board's review. It should be composed of highly aggregated categories that reflect board-formulated financial objectives as well as the organization's key goals and vision.

Getting to Great

- Management should prepare a written rationale describing how the proposed allocation of resources (in broad line-item categories) will lead to achieving board-specified financial objectives.

- The governance-focused budget and rationale should be carefully analyzed by your board's finance committee (and if necessary, sent back to management to be reworked) before being forwarded to your board for its review and approval.

This process effectively subdivides management and governance responsibilities: your board formulates financial objectives, management prepares financial plans designed to achieve them, and then your board assesses the extent to which objectives and budgets are aligned.

PRINCIPLE 30

The board develops a panel of financial indicators, monitors the organization's financial performance, and if problems are detected, demands corrective action.

Board-specified financial objectives and management budgets provide the basis for measuring and monitoring the organization's financial performance and outcomes. For your board to do this, it must develop a set of specific quantitative indicators through roughly the same process it used for quality (Principle 25).

There are three broad types of financial indicators:

- Those specifically keyed to board-formulated *financial objectives.* For example, your board specifies an objective for net operating margin, which then becomes the indicator. Something important enough to be stated as an objective warrants being converted into an indicator, measured, and assessed.

- *Variances* compare operating or budget projections in specific categories with actual results over a period of time, typically a month or a quarter. Some examples are projected versus actual volume (number of admissions or occasions of service), costs or expenses (organization-wide or by program, department, or activity), realized revenue (overall or by service or product category), overtime hours, and number of full-time-equivalent personnel.

- *Ratios* are indexes calculated from the organization's financial statements (balance sheet, revenue and expense statement, cash flow statement) and operating statistics. Standard ratios include *liquidity* (the ability to meet short-term obligations), *activity* (the ability of different types of assets to generate revenue), *capital structure* (the ability to meet long-term obligations), and *profitability* (the ability to generate margins from operations).

A set of financial objective, variance, and ratio indicators should be specified and then periodically monitored and assessed by your board, employing the process described in Chapter Five dealing with the oversight role (Principle 37). These indicators should be continually reviewed by your board's finance committee and periodically by your board. If problems are detected, corrective action by management should be demanded.

PRINCIPLE 31

The board ensures that necessary financial controls are in place.

Your board is accountable for ensuring that accounting systems for supplying accurate and timely information are in place and functioning effectively; transactions are properly authorized, executed, and recorded; and financial statements accurately reflect the organization's financial status. This is accomplished through an annual audit performed for your board by a certified public accounting firm that examines the organization's financial statements; ascertains whether procedures and practices are in accordance with generally accepted accounting principles; assesses the adequacy of financial, accounting, and control systems; and forwards recommendations regarding modifications and improvements to your board and management.

Here's what your board must do:

- Appoint or reappoint the external auditor and approve the audit's scope and approach; the accounting firm performing the audit is retained by your board and is accountable to it, not management.

- Review the auditor's opinion, which presents recommendations for altering systems, procedures, and practices.

- Require management to devise and execute plans to correct any deficiencies.

CHECKUP
Finances

Respond to all items.

	No	Not Entirely	Yes
1. My board understands the importance and nature of its responsibility for ensuring the organization's financial health.	1	2	3
2. My board has formulated a set of key organizational financial objectives.	1	2	3
3. My board ensures that budgets are aligned with key financial objectives.	1	2	3
4. My board has specified a set of financial indicators and employs them to assess the organization's financial health.	1	2	3
5. My board ensures that all necessary financial controls are in place.	1	2	3

Total your responses for the five items, divide by 15, and then multiply by 100. The product is your board's percentage of the maximum score in this area.

Total _____ ÷ 15 × 100 = _____ percent

GETTING STARTED

✓ The single greatest impediment to your board's exercising its responsibility for finances is members who do not possess basic financial literacy. We've found that people often mask their deficiencies in this area and avoid seeking help. Your board must ensure that all members are able to read, understand, and interpret the organization's financial statements. This can be accomplished by an in-service education program (conducted by a member of the organization's finance staff). There are also a number of self-help books designed for those who want a very basic and practical introduction to business finance and accounting.

✓ Begin assuming greater responsibility for finances by formulating financial objectives. Devote a portion of an upcoming meeting to discussing your board's definition of a financially healthy organization. Then specify the most important half-dozen financial objectives the organization must accomplish to be healthy.

✓ Develop an initial set of financial indicators for key objectives, variances, and ratios. Begin with a basic list, and add to it over time.

✓ As a standard practice, we think it is a good idea for the board chairperson to review and approve all organizational disbursements to the CEO (travel, entertainment, and so on). This reinforces accountability and takes pressure off other employees who might find it difficult to question the CEO's expense reports.

✓ After the auditors have presented their opinion and report (typically at a board meeting), make sure your board meets with them in executive session, without the CEO and other management staff present. This gives your board the chance to have a candid conversation with the auditors about the organization's financial practices.

BOARD EFFECTIVENESS AND EFFICIENCY
PRINCIPLE 32

The board is responsible and accountable for itself—its own effectiveness, efficiency, and creativity.

In order to fulfill its responsibilities, your board must have the right governance structure, composition, and infrastructure in place. Principles regarding these aspects of governance will be addressed in Chapters Six, Seven, and Eight.

OTHER FUNCTIONS

This chapter has focused on a set of core responsibilities your board *must* fulfill to meet its obligation to stakeholders. They are functionally necessary and legally mandated under both statutory and case law dealing with a board's duties of loyalty and care.

There are many other tasks your board can and depending on the circumstances should *choose* to do that are not typically considered core responsibilities. Among them are making personal contributions to the organization, participating in fundraising activities, serving as an organizational advocate, and providing advice and counsel to the CEO regarding the execution of his or her managerial role. These are not core governance functions per se because they are not necessary for your board to meet its fiduciary obligation. But they are areas where your board can make significant contributions.

Here are a few thoughts regarding such tasks that your board should consider:

- Board members have the right, and may even be encouraged, to make personal contributions to the organization. However, such contributions should never be the only (or even the most important) prerequisite for being nominated to serve or continuing to serve on the board.

- Board members often have access to potential donors. Because of their commitment to, investment in, and knowledge of the organization, members can be very helpful in soliciting contributions. However, fundraising should be viewed as a supplemental, even peripheral, board activity; it should never overwhelm, displace, or jeopardize your board's fulfilling its core responsibilities. Fundraising is a distinctive organizational function that is often most effectively conducted by a separate foundation with its own board.

- Serving as an advocate for the organization is something that must be expected of all board members. However, they should be very careful speaking for or on behalf of the organization; too many people doing so in an uncoordinated way can send conflicting messages that do more harm than good. When speaking to key external constituents on important issues is necessary, consider having the board chair, accompanied by the CEO, make the presentation.

- CEOs often, quite appropriately, seek counsel from the chair and individual board members on substantive issues related to the performance of their managerial role. Because of their familiarity with the organization (in addition to standing outside of it), members can be very helpful. But the key here is, when providing such counsel, to recognize that members are not acting in a governance capacity, and the advice they provide can be either accepted or rejected.

The overarching notion that flows through all of these recommendations is encapsulated in Principle 33.

PRINCIPLE 33

The defining and fundamental function of a board is governing the organization through fulfilling core responsibilities (for ends, executive performance, quality, finances, and its own effectiveness and efficiency). Board members may be called on to perform other tasks, but if they accept to do so, they are performing discretionary governance activities.

CHAPTER 5

Functioning: Roles

This chapter focuses on the second half of governance functioning, roles—activities your board must perform to fulfill its responsibilities and meet its obligations.

PRINCIPLE 34

The board executes three roles: policy formulation, decision making, and oversight.

If you walk into a meeting of a *great* board (employing principles advanced in Chapter Four) and ask the members what they are doing, the response should be, "We are fulfilling our responsibilities for ends, executive performance, quality, finances, and our own effectiveness and efficiency (self)." But how does a board actually do this? The answer is by performing three roles:

- *Policy formulation*—specifying expectations, directives, and constraints
- *Decision making*—choosing among alternatives regarding matters that require board attention and input
- *Oversight*—monitoring and assessing organizational processes and outcomes

Governance work is a two-sided coin. Fulfilling responsibilities is the what, the substantive aspect of governance; performing roles is the how, activity aspect.

PRINCIPLE 35

The board formulates policies regarding its responsibilities.

Policy formulation is the single best tool your board has to influence the organization, ensuring that it achieves its goals and advances the interests of stakeholders.

A board policy is a declarative statement that directs and constrains subsequent decisions and actions. Policy formulation is the mechanism for performing two absolutely essential governance functions. First, policies express your board's expectations of the organization, management, medical staff and itself. Policies convey what your board wants done (acceptable methods) and accomplished (desired results). Second, policies specify the authority and tasks delegated by your board to management and the medical staff (see Box 5.1).

The most important matters about which your board must formulate policy are its responsibilities (see Box 5.2). Examples of board policies are presented in Appendix A.

Box 5.1. Policy Governance

Our ideas on a board's policy formulation role have been influenced by the work of John Carver. For a more in-depth treatment of policy as a governance tool, we recommend his books:

- *Boards That Make a Difference: A New Design for Leadership in Nonprofit and Public Organizations* (1997)
- *Reinventing Your Board: A Step-by-Step Guide to Implementing Policy Governance* (by John Carver and Miriam Mayhew Carver, 1997)
- *CarverGuide 1: Basic Principles of Policy Governance* (by John Carver and Miriam Mayhew Carver, 1996)

All are published by Jossey-Bass. To order, call (800) 956-7739.

Box 5.2. Policies Regarding Governance Responsibilities

Your board fulfills its responsibilities for ends by formulating policies about

- *Stakeholders*—who they are
- *Vision*—the organization's core purposes and values; what it should become and how it should act, at its very best, in the future
- *Goals*—what must be accomplished to fulfill the vision
- *Alignment*—how management strategies should be linked to goals and the vision

Your board fulfills its responsibility for ensuring high levels of executive performance by formulating policies about

- *Succession*—what should be done when the CEO position becomes vacant
- *Standards*—performance expectations of the CEO
- *Assessment*—the procedures and indicators used to evaluate CEO performance
- *Compensation*—the method employed to adjust the CEO's salary, incentive pay, and benefits
- *Termination*—the circumstances that would necessitate discontinuing the CEO's employment relationship with the organization

Your board fulfills its responsibility for ensuring the quality of care by formulating policies about

- *Definition*—what quality means to your organization
- *Credentialing*—processes and criteria employed to appoint, reappoint, and delineate clinical privileges of the medical staff
- *Indicators and standards*—the criteria employed to assess the quality of care
- *Methods*—the systems that must be in place to monitor and manage quality and utilization
- *Plans*—the types of plans that management and the medical staff must develop to continually improve quality

(Continued)

Box 5.2. Continued

Your board fulfills its responsibility for ensuring the organization's financial health by formulating policies about

- *Financial objectives*—what must be achieved financially to accomplish key organizational goals and fulfill the vision
- *Budgets*—the nature of management's task of devising financial plans and their alignment with board-specified financial objectives, key goals, and the vision
- *Controls*—the procedures that must be in place to ensure that financial statements accurately reflect the organization's financial status and funds are being legitimately disbursed

Your board fulfills its responsibility on self (ensuring its own effectiveness and efficiency), topics addressed in Chapters Six, Seven, and Eight, by formulating policies about

- *Structure*—how governance work will be subdivided and coordinated
- *Composition*—needed board member characteristics, knowledge, skills, experience, and perspectives
- *Infrastructure*—the resources, systems, and procedures required to support the performance of governance work

There are four different types of policies (see Figure 5.1). Your board can convey its expectations and directives by being prescriptive (stating its "thou shalts") or by being prohibitive (stating its "thou shalt nots"). In addition, policies can focus on either results or methods.

Your board may prohibit or prescribe results and methods. However, we have found that the most effective policies prescribe results and prohibit methods. Results are what your board wants accomplished. The best way of conveying such expectations is simply designating them, saying, "Achieve

Figure 5.1. Types of Policies

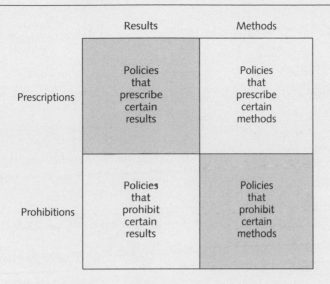

	Results	Methods
Prescriptions	Policies that prescribe certain results	Policies that prescribe certain methods
Prohibitions	Policies that prohibit certain results	Policies that prohibit certain methods

this." As a general rule, your board should avoid specifying methods. There are an infinite number of them; getting involved in determining the way results should be achieved bogs your board down in detail, and prescribing one method eliminates all others. Furthermore, doing so brings your board dangerously close to the line that separates governing from managing. Therefore, if your board has the need to express its expectations regarding methods, we recommend formulating policies that restrict, limit, and prohibit; denoting those that are unacceptable.

Your board's policies should meet all of the following criteria:

- *They should be formulated with great care.* Because your board's policies are among the organization's most important pronouncements, they should be carefully crafted.

- *They should be authoritative.* Policies should be expressed powerfully. Equivocal language (words such as *may, might, should,* and *could*) *must* be avoided. Forcefulness is needed for your board's directives to be understood and heeded.

- *They must be codified.* Policies need to be written for all to see. Otherwise, they are nothing but "hot air." They should also be presented in a common format; Figure 5.2 shows a sample policy form that your board might want to adapt.

- *They should be brief.* Wordiness confuses rather than clarifies. To be understood and have the desired impact, policies must be easily digestible; typically expressed in a page or less.

- *They should be parsimonious.* Here less is more. Your board should formulate as few policies as possible to convey what it expects regarding each of its responsibilities. The noise caused by too many policies obscures what is truly important.

- *They must be comprehensive.* Your board must "weigh in" regarding its most important expectations and directives across the full range of responsibilities, leaving no big gaps. For example, it's ineffective to formulate policies regarding financial objectives without tying them to key goals and the vision.

- *They should be reviewed periodically.* Outmoded and outdated board policies must be tossed out or modified. Nothing depreciates the power and clarity of your board's voice quite so much as policies that have been rendered irrelevant by changed circumstances or the passage of time. We recommend conducting an audit of all board policies every several years, eliminating those that are no longer needed.

PRINCIPLE 36

The board makes decisions regarding matters that require its attention and input.

Ask what the most important things a board does, and the answer is typically: "make decisions." Decisions, like those illustrated in Box 5.3, are important, and your board must make them. However, they should be grounded on, flow from, and be shaped by policy. Your board must first formulate policies regarding key issues in each of its areas of responsibility and

Figure 5.2. Sample Board Policy Form

Responsibility area:

[ ] Ends

[ ] Executive performance

[ ] Quality

[✓] Finances

[ ] Self (governance structure,
composition, and infrastructure)

Policy number: _____10.2_____

Page __1__ of __1__

Date of origination ____10-25-01____

Review: _____every year_____

Issue: criteria to be employed for selecting or reappointing the audit firm

Policy Statement:

_____

_____

_____

_____

_____

_____

_____

_____

_____

_____

_____

_____

then determine what needs to be decided. Otherwise decisions can be idiosyncratic, disjointed, conflicting, and ineffective.

Your board has four options for making decisions:

1. Retaining authority and making decisions itself.

2. Requesting proposals and recommendations from management and the medical staff prior to making a decision.

3. Delegating decision-making authority with constraints; decisions are handed off to management or the medical staff, but with limitations. For example, your board allows the CEO to move funds from one capital budget category to another if they are below a specified dollar amount; if the proposed transfer exceeds this limit, the CEO must seek board approval.

4. Delegating decision making by exception. Management or the medical staff is authorized to make all decisions in a given area, with the exception of those that have been either expressly prohibited or reserved by the board. In the absence of this option, day-to-day operations would come to a standstill.

Here are some suggestions for enhancing your board's decision-making effectiveness:

- Make as few decisions as possible. This somewhat counterintuitive recommendation is consistent with the notion that your board, in executing its roles, should focus first on policy formulation and then on decision making. As you pay more attention to policy and formulate better ones, the number of decisions that have to be made decreases dramatically.

- Do not fall into the trap of ratifying decisions that have been appropriately made by management and the medical staff, for two reasons. First, it wastes a lot of time. Second, when a management or medical staff decision is ratified, it becomes your board's decision, and accountability shifts to the board.

- Due to severe limitations on its time and attention, your board must focus on decisions that matter most in areas where it can add true value. This demands tremendous discipline, as it is easy to become drawn into arenas that may be important but do not require board-level involvement.

- Decision proposals brought forward by management and the medical staff should be reviewed by a board committee before being placed on the agenda for action. Recommendations arrive at the boardroom door as complex, weighty documents with important implications for the organization (if they do not, they should not be put before the board in the first place). On even the very best boards, many members may not have the knowledge, expertise, and experience—or the patience— to evaluate all proposals thoroughly. Consequently, committees must provide "decision-making preparation" by investigating, seeking justification, questioning assumptions, and exploring options prior to the issue's being discussed, deliberated, and acted on by the board.

- Codify all decisions. If they are important enough to be made, they should be written. Board decisions often "slip away," either not captured at all or buried in the minutes. Your board's voice must be recorded in order to convey its directives. Figure 5.3 shows the sort of form that might be used for recording your board's decisions. Decision forms should be consolidated in a ring binder (sorted by responsibility in tabbed sections for each) and periodically distributed to all board members.

• Each year, conduct an audit of your board's decisions. Here are some questions that should be asked:

Were decisions policy-based and consistent?

Were they the types of decisions your board should be making (in terms of their importance and your board's ability to add value)? Did your board have to make these decisions, or could they have been better and more appropriately made by management or the medical staff?

When decisions dealt with proposals made by management or the medical staff, were they thoroughly analyzed by a committee prior to board deliberation and action?

Were they decisions that could have been avoided if a board policy had been in place?

Did any decisions create de facto policies that should have been deliberated and acted on as such?

PRINCIPLE 37

The board oversees (monitors and assesses) key organizational processes and outcomes.

The dashboard of your car does not provide a lot of information, but try driving without it—no gas gauge, speedometer, odometer, battery indicator, oil pressure light, or engine thermometer. Feedback is essential for altering what you do and how well it's done. However, many boards attempt to govern without well-designed dashboards displaying the right gauges. Driving partially blind, they do not have the information they need to determine whether things are working out as planned, promised, and expected.

In executing its oversight role, your board monitors and assesses key organizational processes and outcomes, answering four questions:

Figure 5.3. Sample Board Decision Form

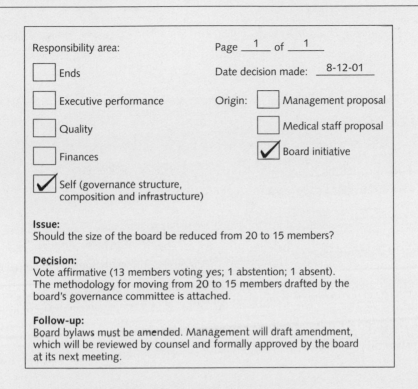

Responsibility area:

☐ Ends

☐ Executive performance

☐ Quality

☐ Finances

☑ Self (governance structure, composition and infrastructure)

Page __1__ of __1__

Date decision made: __8-12-01__

Origin: ☐ Management proposal

☐ Medical staff proposal

☑ Board initiative

Issue:
Should the size of the board be reduced from 20 to 15 members?

Decision:
Vote affirmative (13 members voting yes; 1 abstention; 1 absent).
The methodology for moving from 20 to 15 members drafted by the board's governance committee is attached.

Follow-up:
Board bylaws must be amended. Management will draft amendment, which will be reviewed by counsel and formally approved by the board at its next meeting.

- Is the organization performing in a manner that protects and advances stakeholder interests?

- Are your board's expectations, as conveyed in its policies, being met?

- Are your board's decisions having the desired impact?

- Are your board's directives and constraints being respected as management and the medical staff perform delegated tasks?

As illustrated in Figure 5.4, there are five steps in the board oversight process:

- *Selecting indicators.* There are many things your board could choose to monitor and assess. Where should its attention be focused? What must your board oversee to ensure accountability and obtain the feedback it needs to govern?

- *Specifying standards.* For each indicator, what does your board expect? What constitutes exemplary, adequate, or unacceptable levels of performance?

- *Monitoring results.* For each indicator, gathering data to determine what actually happened.

- *Assessing* what was achieved in light of what was expected.

- *Taking action.* What should be done if there is a difference between the standard and the result for a particular indicator?

Box 5.4 provides several illustrations of this process.

Your board must take the initiative in specifying the type of information it needs to perform its oversight role effectively. Although management and the medical staff must be involved (providing perspective, expertise, and data), this responsibility rests squarely with your board; only your board can determine which indicators and standards are needed to oversee in a manner that ensures accountability.

Figure 5.4. The Board Oversight Process

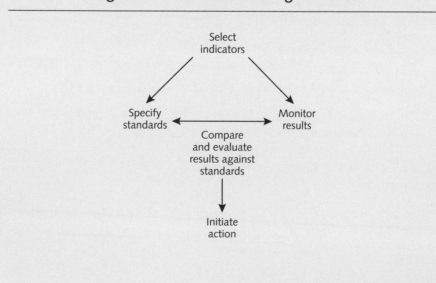

Box 5.4. Some Illustrations of the Board Oversight Process

Indicator: Inpatient medication error rate

Standard: x percent of the number of medications administered

Result: x percent

Comparison: Target not met

Action: Request analysis and plan from the quality improvement department (working with the medical staff quality committee) to be presented at board meeting on (*date*)

Indicator: Nonexempt employee turnover

Standard: Less than x percent of adjusted full-time-equivalent employees per year

Result: x percent for the most recent year

Comparison: Standard exceeded

Action: Reward and celebrate

Indicator: Net operating margin

Standard: x percent

Result: x percent (annually adjusted) for the last six months of the present fiscal year; performance x percent under target

Comparison: Standard not met

Action: Management analysis and plan to enhance revenues and reduce costs to be presented at the next meeting of the board finance committee; net operating margin report and analysis to be forwarded to the board monthly (rather than quarterly, as in the past)

Indicator: Average board meeting attendance rate

Standard: Not to exceed x percent (both excused and unexcused absences)

(Continued)

What dashboards are needed? We recommend five, one for each board responsibility. At a minimum, a set of "gauges" (indicators and associated standards) must be developed for each:

- *Ends*—to determine whether the vision is being fulfilled, goals are being accomplished, and key strategies are being effectively pursued

- *Executive performance*—to determine whether the CEO's performance is in line with board expectations

- *Quality*—to determine whether the quality of care is at the desired level

- *Finances*—to determine whether the organization's financial performance meets board expectations

- *Board effectiveness and efficiency*—to determine whether your board is performing appropriately and creatively and making a positive contribution

Here are some guidelines for designing board oversight dashboards:

- If something is important enough for your board to express an expectation about (through a policy statement), it warrants being monitored and assessed.

- If your board attempts to monitor and assess too many things, it will oversee nothing particularly well. We suggest that no more than a dozen gauges be developed for each board responsibility.

- A standard must be attached to each indicator, specifying levels of unacceptable, adequate, and exemplary performance. That is, your board's most important expectations (conveyed in its policies) drive the selection of both indicators and standards. For example, consider a board policy regarding overall financial performance: "The net margin from operations must exceed x percent." The indicator is the net margin from operations; the standard is x percent.

- Indicators must be quantifiable. If something is not measurable, it cannot be monitored. However, it's important to keep in mind that most subjective performance indicators can be quantified. For example, employee satisfaction (inherently subjective) can be measured by an appropriately designed questionnaire.

- Remember that data become information only when they are organized. We've found that the best method is graphical. A graph is worth a

Figure 5.5. A Graphical Approach to Oversight Reporting

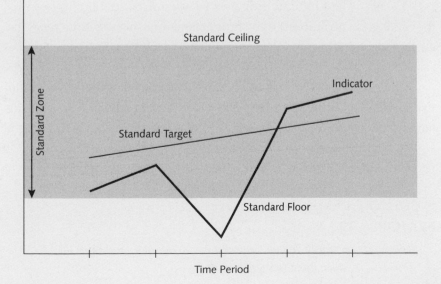

thousand words (or columns of numbers). Figure 5.5 illustrates a format that we have found useful.

Picture your board's dashboard system as a three-ring binder with five dividers labeled for each of your board's responsibilities. Behind each divider there are about a dozen sheets of paper, each tracking a different indicator and conveying an associated standard (portrayed as in Figure 5.5) selected by your board to measure and assess its most important expectations.

PRINCIPLE 38

When it meets, the board spends the vast majority of its time executing roles; formulating policy, making decisions, and overseeing.

How much of your board meeting time is spent passively listening—to background information, briefings, presentations, and reports from management, medical staff, consultants, and the board's own committees? We estimate that the figure exceeds 60 percent for most boards. Listening is important. But could your board really govern, make a difference, and add value if it spent 100 percent of its time just listening? The answer is clearly no.

One of the best indicators of a board's performance (and its potential for making a contribution) is the proportion of its meeting time spent discussing, deliberating, and debating policies, decisions, and oversight parameters regarding its responsibilities.

Figure 5.6 depicts a distribution of effort that we consider optimal. Notice that total meeting time is 80 percent role-related activity, 15 percent listening, and 5 percent non-role-related activity (socializing, downtime, and so on). Fifty percent of role-related activity is spent formulating policy, 30 percent engaged in oversight, and 20 percent making decisions.

PRINCIPLE 39

The board acts only collectively, never individually; and once an action is agreed to, members support it.

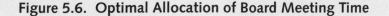

Figure 5.6. Optimal Allocation of Board Meeting Time

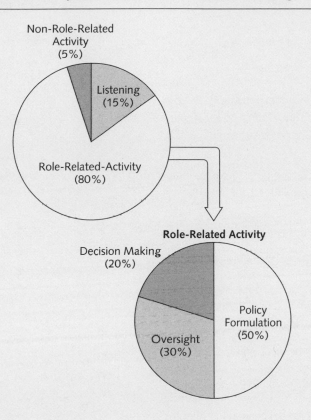

Governance is a team sport. When your board acts, it must do so together. Individual members have absolutely no power; board authority derives from the group as a whole. Members should argue, deliberate, debate, and disagree with one another regarding a particular issue when it is being discussed. But after the vote is taken, members must lock arms and support your board's decision even if they were against it. Divisiveness depreciates the quality and clarity of your board's voice. When a member finds himself or herself continually unable to support your board's collective will, it is time for that member to resign.

CHECKUP
Roles

Respond to all items.

	No	Not Entirely	Yes
1. My board understands that its core roles are formulating policy, making decisions, and overseeing.	1	2	3
2. My board formulates policies regarding its responsibilities.	1	2	3
3. My board makes decisions regarding matters that require its attention and input.	1	2	3
4. My board oversees (monitors and assesses) key organizational processes and outcomes.	1	2	3
5. In meetings, my board spends the majority of time performing its roles; formulating policy, making decisions, and overseeing.	1	2	3
6. My board acts only collectively; once we act, members support our board's policies and decisions.	1	2	3

Total your responses for the six items, divide by 18, and then multiply by 100. The product is your board's percentage of the maximum score in this area.

Total _____ ÷ 18 × 100 = _____ percent

GETTING STARTED

 If your board has not been explicitly employing policy formulation as a governance tool, begin doing so immediately. The best way to start is framing major issues on which your board must act as proposed policies. The nature and substance of the policy are discussed and voted on by your board at its meetings. Consider employing a policy form like the one in Figure 5.2.

 Most boards have adopted policies in one form or another, but they are recorded in meeting minutes. Scan your minutes for the most important policy statements, put them in the form suggested here, and then have the board reconsider and act on them.

 Over the next year, your board should spend a portion of each meeting deliberating its most important expectations in each area of responsibility (ends, executive performance, quality, finances, and board effectiveness and efficiency). The discussions should then prompt the drafting of policies that convey these expectations.

 Examine your minutes over the past several years, and conduct an audit of your board's decisions. Codify the decisions identified employing a form like the one presented in Figure 5.3. Using the form, present them to the board for review, ratifying, modifying, and reversing decisions where appropriate.

 Develop initial oversight dashboards for each area of responsibility. Initially, focus on designing about a half-dozen gauges (indicators and associated standards) for each. The place to begin is your board's most important expectations as conveyed in its policies.

OVERALL BOARD FUNCTIONING

Chapters Four and Five have focused on principles about board functioning; the responsibilities your board must fulfill, and the roles it must perform to govern properly. How your board chooses to function—the way it allocates its precious attention, time, and effort—more than any other factor, will determine its performance and contributions.

PRINCIPLE 40

The board has a coherent, precise, shared, and empowering notion of the type of work it must do, its responsibilities, and its roles.

Your board's description of its functions should be codified in a charter, incorporating the principles put forth in Chapters Four and Five. An illustration is provided in Box 5.5.

Box 5.5. A Typical Board Charter

Our board's ultimate obligation is to ensure that the organization's resources and capacities are deployed in a manner that advances and protects stakeholder interests. To function as the stakeholders' agent and add value to the organization on their behalf, we *formulate policy* (convey expectations, direct, and guide), *make decisions* (choose among alternatives), and *oversee* (monitor and assess) the organization's ends, executive performance, quality of care, and finances, in addition to our board's effective and efficient performance and contributions. The nature of our board's work is defined by its responsibilities and roles.

Our board is responsible for determining the organization's *ends*. To fulfill this responsibility, we

- Formulate the organization's vision, its core values and purposes
- Specify key goals that, if accomplished, lead to the vision being fulfilled
- Ensure that strategies developed by management are aligned with key goals and the vision

Our board is responsible for ensuring high levels of *executive performance*. To fulfill this responsibility, we

---

- Select and recruit the chief executive officer (CEO)
- Specify CEO performance objectives
- Assess the CEO's performance and contributions
- Adjust the CEO's compensation package
- Should the need arise, terminate the CEO's employment with the organization

Subject to its directives and oversight, the board delegates all management functions to the CEO. The CEO is the only employee directly accountable to the board.

Our board is responsible for ensuring the *quality of care* provided in and by the organization. To fulfill this responsibility, we

- Define quality
- Appoint, reappoint, and delineate privileges of medical staff members
- Ensure that necessary quality and utilization monitoring systems are in place and functioning effectively
- Determine quality standards and employ them periodically to assess the care provided
- Ensure that the organization has developed a plan to continually improve quality

Our board is responsible for the organization's *financial health*, protecting and enhancing the community's investment in it. To fulfill this responsibility, we

- Establish financial objectives
- Ensure that planning and budgeting are undertaken by management in a manner that meets our financial objectives
- Monitor and assess financial performance and outcomes
- Ensure that necessary control mechanisms are in place

(Continued)

Box 5.5. Continued

We are responsible for our *self,* our board's own effectiveness, efficiency, and creativity. Our board ensures

- That it discharges core governance responsibilities and roles in ways that advance stakeholder interests and adds value to the organization
- That its structure is appropriate
- That its members possess the needed characteristics, knowledge, skills, and experiences to govern
- That the necessary resources and systems are in place to assist us in performing our work

CHAPTER 6

Structure

Structure is the "anatomical" aspect of governance; it provides the context for and significantly affects your board's functioning, composition, and infrastructure. Several structural issues are key:

- Centralization or decentralization of governance
- In a decentralized structure, number of boards and division and coordination of governance work among them
- Board size
- Board committees: number, types, and functions

Because a health care organization can be composed of "parent" and multiple subsidiary corporations, governance structure can be either centralized or decentralized.

In a centralized structure, as illustrated in Figure 6.1, the organization is governed by a single board. If it is composed of separately incorporated subsidiary organizations, they do not have boards of their own.

A decentralized governance structure (see Figure 6.2) has two key characteristics: the organization is composed of one or more separately incorporated subsidiary organizations, and these subsidiaries have their own boards. The parent board exercises ultimate authority over subsidiary boards, but governance responsibilities and roles are divided among them and coordinated.

Figure 6.1. Centralized Governance Structure

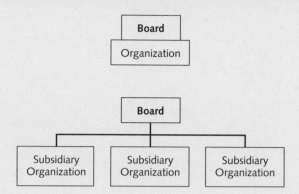

Decentralized governance in some form is the norm in the health care industry. It is estimated that over 65 percent of hospitals are either part of a system or have subsidiary corporations.

PRINCIPLE 41

The board recognizes the importance of governance structure. This structure is consciously designed on the basis of explicit principles, criteria, and choices.

Structure matters. A poorly designed structure will impair your board; an appropriate one will facilitate effective and efficient performance of gover-

Figure 6.2. Decentralized Governance Structure

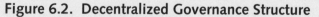

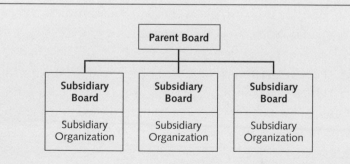

Getting to Great

nance work, although structure alone cannot guarantee this. In addition, efforts to implement principles regarding board composition and infrastructure will be aided by a good structure and impeded by a poor one.

Design of the organization's governance structure should be guided by the following criteria:

- *Intentionally.* An appropriate, efficient structure is not accidental. It is the product of careful analysis and explicit choices. Recognize that structure must be consciously designed by your board.

- *Functionality.* Function should determine form, not the other way around. Structure must be crafted to support and facilitate fulfilling responsibilities and performing roles.

- *Adaptability.* Structure should not be set in stone. Rather, it should be viewed as a flexible or even temporary vehicle that will be periodically modified as circumstances and needs change.

- *Individuality.* Structure should be customized to the distinctive characteristics of the organization and the particular governance challenges it faces.

PRINCIPLE 42

Governance structure is streamlined.

Here, less is more, and simplicity is better. Parsimony should drive the design process, aiming for as few "moving parts" as necessary.

Streamlined structure aids in focusing and efficiently deploying your board's effort; an overweight and cumbersome structure typically diffuses and squanders it. Furthermore, a poor structure consumes an inordinately large amount of valuable executive time. Every board and committee meeting must be staffed, prepared for, attended, documented, and followed up.

All else being equal, the most effective and efficient structure has the fewest number of governance layers, boards, board members, and committees; it is no larger and no more complex than is necessary to facilitate performance of the organization's governance work.

PRINCIPLE 43

In a multicorporate organizational form, the parent or system board makes an explicit choice regarding whether to employ a centralized or decentralized governance structure after carefully weighing the benefits and costs of each alternative.

Many governance experts recommend that health care systems should move from decentralized toward centralized structures. Circumstances and needs vary, and the pros and cons of each option depend on them.

Centralized Structure

Potential Pros

More complete governance integration, prompting and providing the platform for greater "systemness" in management and clinical operations

More rapid governance decision making

Greater focus on systemwide issues

Fewer resources and less management time spent on governance

Greater board expertise and experience (since fewer members must be recruited)

Potential Cons

Disconnection of parent board from the circumstances, challenges, and operations of subsidiary organizations

Decentralized Structure

Potential Pros

Greater sensitivity to local community, organizational, and medical staff issues

Governance workload shared among multiple boards

Possibility of developing specialized governance functions (for example, where subsidiary hospital board focuses on credentialing and quality-of-care issues)

A larger cadre of organizational advocates due to the larger number of boards and board members

Potential Cons

Slower governance metabolism, as significant initiatives move through multiple layers and boards

Increased conflict due to lack of clarity or consensus or differences among boards regarding their authority and power

Here are some recommendations your board might want to entertain:

• Construct a chart of the organization's governance structure: all incorporated entities owned or controlled, in whole or in part, by the organization and their relationships and all boards of owned or wholly or partially controlled organizations and their relationships (see Figure 6.3). Members are often surprised at just how many separately incorporated entities and boards the organization actually has. Redesign must begin with an accurate description.

• Attempt to reduce the number of separately incorporated entities within the organization. Over the past several decades (because of the need to maximize reimbursement, enter new markets, and limit liability), many health care provider organizations have undergone massive subsidiary proliferation. Changes in laws, regulations, and circumstances have eliminated the need for maintaining many of these entities. Fewer corporations will necessitate fewer boards.

• In a system with all or most of its assets deployed in one market, decentralized governance is very difficult to justify. In such cases, particularly when the medical staffs of separate hospitals can be consolidated, the advantages of centralized governance should be carefully considered.

• Where the assets of a system are spread across a number of geographically dispersed markets, some type of decentralized governance is probably the only reasonable alternative.

• Some subsidiaries must be separately incorporated and have their own boards due to legal requirements—examples (in most states) are health plans, for-profit organizations, and (in some cases) medical groups.

• Foundations should typically have their own boards. The reason is that a foundation board's job is one part governing and two parts raising money. Melding these different purposes in one board requires distinctive functions, structure, composition, and infrastructure (see Box 6.1).

Where decentralized governance is warranted, certain structural options can minimize complexity and reduce the number of board members needed. Subsidiary organizations can be governed by any of the following:

Figure 6.3. A Typical Governance Chart

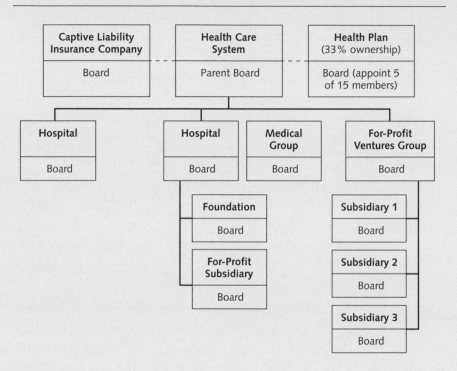

- *Mirror boards.* The parent board serves as the board of a subsidiary organization. Structurally and legally, there are two boards; in terms of membership, there is only one. A single group of individuals simultaneously does the "governance business" of two organizations.

- *Interlocking board membership.* Some members of the parent board hold some (but not all) seats on a subsidiary board.

- *Internal (management) boards.* The board of a subsidiary organization is composed entirely or primarily of management team members from the parent organization.

There are challenges associated with each of these options (see Box 6.2).

PRINCIPLE 44

In organizations employing a decentralized governance structure, the parent board has systems in place to monitor subsidiary organization and board performance.

In organizations with multiple boards, the parent board still bears ultimate responsibility, authority, and accountability for subsidiaries and their governance. Accordingly, and consistent with performance of a board's oversight role (Principle 37):

- The parent board should develop and periodically monitor a set of strategic, operational, and financial indicators and standards that reflect subsidiary organization performance and outcomes. Because subsidiaries can have very different purposes, characteristics, and challenges, indicators should be customized for each.

Box 6.2. Challenges Associated with Alternative Decentralized Governance Structures

Mirror Boards

- To fulfill legal requirements, the different boards must hold separate meetings and keep separate minutes.
- The distinction in responsibilities and roles between the boards can become confused.
- The attention and effort dedicated to one board (typically the subsidiary) can be slighted.
- The workload of individuals, who must serve on two boards simultaneously, is increased.

For these reasons, we recommend that only one mirror board be configured for a given parent.

Interlocking Membership

This option might decrease, albeit slightly, the total number of board members in a system but does not offer much structural simplification. It does, however, provide one way to coordinate the functioning of a parent and subsidiary boards. And since different sets of parent board members can be "interlocked" across different subsidiary boards, it has much broader applicability than the creation of a mirror board.

Internal (Management) Boards

- If the subsidiary board governs a nonprofit organization, IRS regulations prohibit management or other insiders from holding more than 49 percent of the seats. Thus this option is available only to for-profit subsidiaries.
- This arrangement blurs the distinction between governance and management obligations and functions. In addition, subsidiary executives wind up reporting managerially to exactly the same group to whom they are accountable for governance. One must question what value, if any, is added through such an arrangement.

- Annually, the parent board should request from each subsidiary board a report detailing its key challenges, strengths, weaknesses, and any specific initiatives that are being undertaken to improve governance performance and contributions.

If the organization has a large number of subsidiaries, we recommend forming a special committee to assist the parent board in executing this important oversight role (see Principle 37 in Chapter Five). In addition, subsidiary board self-assessments (see Principle 72 in Chapter Eight) should be reviewed periodically.

PRINCIPLE 45

Unless there are compelling reasons to do otherwise, a board should have between nine and nineteen members.

Board size is a fundamental and critical structural characteristic that has a significant effect on all aspects of governance functioning, composition, and infrastructure. Thus board size should be based on an explicit rationale and subject to periodic review.

Very large boards are often carryovers from times past when their primary purpose was philanthropic. Today, other than for foundations, the central obligation of boards is governing, not fundraising. Thus having a large number of members for this purpose is no longer necessary. Other common reasons given for having a large board include providing an opportunity for significant stakeholder involvement in governance and being able to spread an overly burdensome amount of board work (a symptom of ineffective governance in itself) among many members.

Large boards have several strikes against them. First, they are more cumbersome deliberative and decision-making bodies than smaller ones. Second, because of this, they tend to have active and powerful executive committees, where the real work is done. This frequently creates a two-class system, leaving members who are not on the executive committee feeling disenfranchised. Third, very large boards tend to reduce the involvement of individual members, thereby decreasing their commitment. Finally, big boards tend to have more and larger committees simply to guarantee that every member has an opportunity to serve on several of them.

Very small boards have several significant disadvantages as well. First, they do not have enough members to provide needed diversity of characteristics, knowledge, skills, experience, and perspectives. Second, one or two members can dominate the board and exert disproportionate influence. Third, the absence of a few members can dramatically affect their ability to get work done at board meetings. Fourth, an unexpected departure of a talented member can be very disruptive due to a lack of "bench strength." Fifth, such boards often demand too much of their members and run the risk of burning them out.

While one specific size is not best for all boards, there is an optimal range. Boards that fall outside it, being either too large or small, seriously compromise their effectiveness, efficiency, and creativity. Your board should be large enough to get the work done and achieve a requisite amount of diversity yet small enough to function as a cohesive, focused, deliberative policy formulation, decision-making, and oversight body.

Our experience, in addition to the group dynamics and performance literature, suggests that the optimal board size is nine to nineteen members. This range should be the "default setting." If your board decides to be either smaller or larger, it should have a carefully thought out, explicit, and persuasive rationale for doing so. Furthermore, we recommend that your board be composed of an odd number of members to minimize the possibility of tie votes on controversial issues.

Board size in subsidiary organizations, where a decentralized governance structure is employed, is often (and quite appropriately) either above or below the optimal nine-to-nineteen-member range due to their functions. For example, a subsidiary organization board may have a very narrow set of tasks delegated to it by the parent. In such instances, fewer members might be needed. Similarly, a subsidiary foundation (fundraising) board might be very large in order to maximize community liaison and member giving in addition to supplying a "workforce" to solicit funds from others. But the overarching principle still applies: you must have a compelling reason for constructing a board outside the optimal range. The rationale should be explicitly tied to the board's purpose and designed to optimize its functioning. It is important to remember that subsidiary organization boards are, first and foremost, governing bodies. They have important obligations, functions, and legal duties to fulfill that are impaired when their size is inappropriate.

PRINCIPLE 46

In decentralized structures, the authority, responsibilities, and roles of parent and subsidiary boards are explicitly and precisely specified.

Health care organizations with decentralized structures face a unique challenge: governance work must be effectively and efficiently divided and coordinated among parent and subsidiary boards. When this is done poorly, significant problems can arise: policy formulation, decision making, and oversight take more time; rework increases; and conflict arises over the authority and functions of different boards.

In organizations with decentralized governance structures, board work must be explicitly and precisely mapped (see Figure 6.4), specifying how responsibilities and roles are partitioned. There are three options: a specific role (policy formulation, decision making, and oversight) with respect to a given responsibility (ends, executive performance, quality, finances, and board effectiveness and efficiency) can be

- *Retained* by the parent board
- *Shared* by the parent and subsidiary boards
- *Delegated* (with or without constraints) to the subsidiary boards

See Box 6.3 for some illustrations.

PRINCIPLE 47

If advisory bodies are employed, their functions are clearly specified and differentiated from those of governing boards.

Figure 6.4. Board Work Mapping in Decentralized Governance Structures

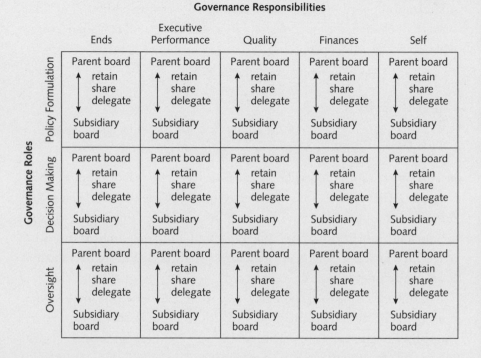

Governance Responsibilities

		Ends	Executive Performance	Quality	Finances	Self
Governance Roles	Policy Formulation	Parent board ↑ retain share ↓ delegate Subsidiary board	Parent board ↑ retain share ↓ delegate Subsidiary board	Parent board ↑ retain share ↓ delegate Subsidiary board	Parent board ↑ retain share ↓ delegate Subsidiary board	Parent board ↑ retain share ↓ delegate Subsidiary board
	Decision Making	Parent board ↑ retain share ↓ delegate Subsidiary board	Parent board ↑ retain share ↓ delegate Subsidiary board	Parent board ↑ retain share ↓ delegate Subsidiary board	Parent board ↑ retain share ↓ delegate Subsidiary board	Parent board ↑ retain share ↓ delegate Subsidiary board
	Oversight	Parent board ↑ retain share ↓ delegate Subsidiary board	Parent board ↑ retain share ↓ delegate Subsidiary board	Parent board ↑ retain share ↓ delegate Subsidiary board	Parent board ↑ retain share ↓ delegate Subsidiary board	Parent board ↑ retain share ↓ delegate Subsidiary board

Many health care organizations have entities called "advisory boards." This is a misnomer because they do not bear legal fiduciary responsibility for the organization and hence do not govern. However, advisory bodies can often behave as if they do. In such situations, conflict arises between them and the "real" board.

If your organization has an advisory body, its purposes and functions should be clearly defined, perhaps along the following lines:

- Providing input to the governing board or management and serving as a "sounding board" for it; the advice offered may be either accepted or rejected.
- Providing a link to the organization's stakeholders and customers
- Serving as an organizational advocate in the community

Box 6.3. Division of Responsibility Among Parent and Subsidiary Boards

CEO Selection in Subsidiary Organizations

Responsibility of the parent-organization CEO with input and advice provided by the subsidiary board.

Specifying Subsidiary-Organization Financial Objectives

Developed by the subsidiary board based on policies formulated by the parent board; subsidiary board financial objectives must be aligned with and contribute to accomplishing those specified by the parent.

Quality Oversight in Subsidiary Organizations

Indicators and standards specified by the parent board; monitoring and assessment conducted by the subsidiary board with biannual reports to the parent.

Subsidiary Board Composition

Subsidiary boards recruit and nominate new board members based on criteria specified by the parent; such members must be recommended to the parent for approval.

PRINCIPLE 48

The board specifies the functions of its committees.

Few boards can function without committees. They are needed because board meetings do not generally provide enough time to get all the work done, many issues can be better addressed by groups smaller than the board, and committees can tap needed expertise by including individuals as members who do not serve on the board.

A key issue for your board is determining how work should be divided and coordinated (between the board and its committees and among these committees) in a way that facilitates effective and efficient governance but does not compromise your board's integrity, authority, or responsibility.

Committees cannot be expected to fulfill responsibilities and perform roles that are your board's alone and should never be allowed to do so. The legal and fiduciary obligation to govern rests with your board, not its committees. With the possible exception of an executive committee, they have no authority and should never formulate policies or make decisions. Their appropriate role is supporting and facilitating your board when it meets by performing "governance staff work." Committees do this by undertaking analyses and framing recommendations that serve as the basis of your board's discussions, deliberations, and actions.

PRINCIPLE 49

The number and types of committees are specifically designed to aid the board in fulfilling its responsibilities.

Your board must resolve two basic questions regarding committees: Which committees should it have? What should they do?

Many boards have a "standing" committee structure, which does not change from year to year. This rigid arrangement runs the risk of freezing board focus and functioning while the circumstances the organization faces evolve and change. Such boards often struggle to effectively address new issues with an increasingly outmoded committee structure.

The challenge is to have an effective and efficient committee structure that is relevant to current conditions (which change from year to year) and reflect your board's responsibilities (which do not).

The solution is for your board to regularly tailor its committee structure and the functioning of each committee to established needs and priorities. This can be accomplished through a zero-based committee design process.

Zero-based design forces your board to reevaluate its committees every year. At the end of each year, all committees are automatically dissolved. Your board then determines which, if any, of the previous year's committees should be reestablished and which new ones should be created. Only once organizational challenges and board objectives have been specified can your board appropriately determine what committees, if any, it should have.

Boards employing a zero-based design typically find that several committees continue to exist from year to year—the ones that support fulfilling of core governance responsibilities—under various names such as these:

- Executive committee
- Vision and goals (or "ends") committee
- Executive performance and compensation committee
- Quality committee
- Finance committee
- Governance committee

Much of the value of the zero-based approach is that it forces your board to critically and explicitly assess the contribution made by and the need for each committee, taking none for granted. This generally produces changes in committee structure in addition to modification of individual committee charters, objectives, and work plans (see Principle 50).

Because the committees of most boards are specified in the bylaws, any alteration in committee structure would require annual amendments of the bylaws. Since this would be excessively burdensome, we recommend a one-time bylaws revision stating that the board employs a zero-based design process, configuring its committees at the beginning of each year.

Committee design should be guided by the following criteria:

- *Authority.* Only the board bears ultimate responsibility for governing the organization. Board committees, except in very proscribed and infrequent situations (such as an executive committee that can act in emergencies), have no independent authority to decide or act on behalf of the full board.
- *Minimalism.* The fewest possible number of board committees are to be created in any given year.
- *Functionality.* Committees are established for the purpose of assisting the board in fulfilling its responsibilities and performing its roles.

PRINCIPLE 50

The objectives, functions, and tasks of committees are specified by the board.

Your board must do more than determine what committees it will have and specify their functions; it must also direct them. Committees lacking focus can pull your board in many different directions at once, hindering effective governance.

Although each committee performs different functions and tasks, the sum total of these activities must converge to move your board toward the achievement of its annual governance objectives (see Principle 65 in Chapter Eight).

Your board should begin framing, directing and constraining the work of its committees through the formulation of charters specifying committee objectives and key functions. Examples of committee charters are provided in Appendix B.

Committee functioning should be specified and fine-tuned by requiring each committee to develop an annual work plan that is reviewed by the executive committee and approved by your board. Work plans explicitly describe the key priorities, tasks, "deliverables," and deadlines of each committee. Such plans focus a committee's efforts on important work it must perform on behalf of your board. In addition, they provide a basis for assessing committee performance and contributions at the end of each year.

PRINCIPLE 51

Governance structure is thoroughly assessed, and modified if necessary, on a regular basis.

Regular evaluation is essential for ensuring that governance structure is appropriate, effective, and efficient. Such an evaluation addresses questions such as these:

• What aspects of governance structure are working well? Which should be working better?

- What aspects of structure are in place and have not been eliminated or modified just because "we have always done it that way"?

- What structural alterations (layers of governance, number of boards, board size, number and types of committees) are needed to govern more effectively and efficiently?

Most evaluations of governance structure are conducted annually or biannually as part of a more comprehensive board self-assessment process (see Principle 72 in Chapter Eight).

CHECKUP
Structure

Respond to only items that are relevant to your organization and your board.

	No	Not Entirely	Yes
1. My board recognizes the importance of governance structure and intentionally designs it on the basis of careful analysis, precise criteria, and explicit choices.	1	2	3
2. The organization's governance structure is streamlined; it has the smallest possible number of governance layers, boards, board committees, and members.	1	2	3
3. If the organization is composed of more than one separately incorporated entity, the parent board has made an explicit choice (based on careful analysis) whether to employ a centralized or decentralized governance structure.	1	2	3

4. My board's size falls within the range   1   3
   of nine to nineteen members.

5. If your organization has a decentralized   1   2   3
   governance structure, the authority,
   responsibilities, and roles of parent
   and subsidiary boards are explicitly
   and precisely specified.

6. If advisory bodies are employed, their   1   2   3
   functions are clearly specified and
   differentiated from those of the
   governing board.

7. My board has the appropriate   1   2   3
   number and types of committees
   needed to support and facilitate
   its work.

8. The authority of committees   1   2   3
   vis-à-vis my board is precisely
   specified; the board governs,
   and committees do "governance
   staff work."

9. Charters specifying key objectives,   1   2   3
   functions, and duties have been
   developed for all board committees.

10. Board's committees are required to   1   2   3
    develop annual work plans.

11. Governance structure is thoroughly   1   2   3
    assessed, and modified if necessary,
    on a regular basis.

Total your responses. Count the number of items to which you responded, and multiply it by 3. Divide this number into your total score, and

112

then multiply by 100. The product is your board's percentage of the maximum score in this area.

Total _____ ÷ (number of items scored _____ × 3 = _____) × 100 = _____ percent

GETTING STARTED

✓ Allocate some time at an upcoming board meeting to briefly review your governance structure. Are the principles advanced in this chapter being employed?

✓ Prepare a governance organizational chart, identifying all boards and board committees and their reporting relationships.

✓ Review and evaluate the size of your board. Is the present number of members justified? Does the present size either facilitate or impair the way governance work is performed or how well it is performed? Should the size of your board be modified?

✓ Undertake an initial zero-based committee design activity. Evaluate the need for each committee in terms of helping your board fulfill its core responsibilities and roles and dealing with critical organizational challenges requiring board input.

✓ Draft charters for each board committee, specifying their key objectives, functions, scope of work, and tasks.

CHAPTER 7

Composition

C omposition deals with the most basic aspect of governance: board members and what they bring into the boardroom (see Box 7.1).

All boards have a composition model (typically specified in the organization's charter or bylaws). There are three types:

- *Elected*—board members are chosen by a vote of the organization's stakeholders. The key here is that stakeholders, or their representatives, directly select board members.

- *Appointed*—board members are chosen by some other entity: a parent board (in a multilayered governance structure as described in Chapter Six), sponsoring organization, or governmental agency. Here control of the board's composition rests outside the organization.

- *Self-selected*—the board nominates and chooses its own members.

These models can be combined in various ways. For example, a board can nominate its own members (self-selected model), but a parent board must approve the slate (appointed model); or some members may be appointed and others elected directly.

While each model imposes different constraints, the elected and appointed options severely restrict a board's ability to design and manage its own composition. Accordingly, many of the principles presented here are best applied when members are: selected by the board itself or nominated

Box 7.1. Casting

At a film festival, a young student approached the famous director John Huston and challenged him: "The critics contend, Mr. Huston, that 50 percent of the success of your movies is due entirely to casting." Huston replied, "They're wrong, my young friend. It's *all* casting."

The story may be apocryphal, but Huston clearly had an appreciation that casting decisions—choosing who plays which parts—is critical to success. The same is true for your board.

Pause for a moment and reflect on your board's casting—its composition.

- How are new board members chosen? Is a carefully designed methodology employed? Are explicit criteria used to seek out, screen, and select members, based on organizational challenges and board needs?

- How many underperforming members does your board have? Who are they? Why are they allowed to continue serving?

- Which members make the greatest contributions? What distinctive competencies or capacities do they bring to your board?

- What are your board's compositional strengths; knowledge, skills, experience, perspectives, and values?

- What are your board's compositional weaknesses, its competency and capacity gaps?

- Have any members ever been removed for poor performance or a lack of contribution?

- Why were you selected as a member of this board? What talents did you bring? Have you fulfilled your promise?

- Overall, how would you rate the quality of your board's casting?

by the board and subject to election or ratification by some other body (for example, a health system parent board).

PRINCIPLE 52

The board consciously and proactively designs and manages its composition.

No other single factor so directly affects your board's performance and contributions as its composition. The quality of your board and its ability to govern depend on the characteristics, knowledge, skills, experience, perspectives, and values of its members.

It is impossible for your board to design its composition without being absolutely clear regarding its obligations, responsibilities, and roles (the focus of Chapters Three, Four, and Five). A board that does not know what it is supposed to do cannot determine the types of individuals needed to do it.

To design and manage its composition, your board must

- Identify, screen, and select new board members, making sure that their characteristics, competencies, and experience are aligned with organizational and board needs
- Orient new members
- Specify member expectations
- Develop board members
- Periodically assess the performance and contributions of individual members
- Ensure an appropriate balance between inside or ex officio and outside members

PRINCIPLE 53

Members are recruited and selected on the basis of explicit criteria as part of a board profiling process.

Many boards deal with composition issues idiosyncratically and opportunistically. A seat becomes available, and an acquaintance of a present member or the CEO is selected, with little attention paid to board needs or investigation of the candidate's potential to make a contribution.

Great board casting begins with a carefully designed, criteria-based system that is used to identify, screen, and select new members.

Although the specific criteria will vary, the categories should not. We recommend four (see Box 7.2):

- *Basic qualifications*—baseline attributes every candidate must possess to be considered for board membership. They should be uniformly applied, with no exceptions. For example, it would not make sense to put an intelligent and otherwise well-qualified person on your board who is unable to attend most meetings.

- *Demographic characteristics*—dealing with such things as place of residence, community involvement, age, gender, and ethnicity. They are applied as general guidelines to achieve a mix of characteristics across board members.

- *General competencies*—knowledge, skills, and experience a candidate must possess to become a high-performing and contributing member.

- *Special competencies*—specific talents needed by your board to address its challenges and opportunities. They are variably applied to members with different but complementary skills and experience; some, but not all, board members must possess them.

The process of identifying and deliberating specific criteria forces your board to be explicit and precise about the member characteristics and capacities it needs.

A case-by-case application of criteria can, however, still result in your board's lacking the appropriate mix of attributes. Therefore, we recommend that a criteria-based approach be employed in conjunction with a board profiling process (see Figure 7.1), which entails the following steps:

1. Employ specific basic, demographic, general, and special competency

Box 7.2. Member Screening and Selection Criteria

These criteria are not recommendations; they are examples intended to stimulate and focus your board's thinking and deliberation.

Basic Qualifications

- Willingness to serve on the board
- Commitment to and interest in the organization (its vision, mission, and key goals)
- Ability to meet time and effort requirements (board and committee meeting preparation and attendance, educational activities, retreats, organizational events)
- High level of personal and professional integrity

Demographic Characteristics

- Percentage of board members who must live or work in the organization's service area
- Minimum and maximum age requirements
- Diversity expectations and targets regarding gender, age, race, and ethnicity

General Competencies

- Intelligence
- Ability to articulate ideas and positions clearly
- Capacity to work productively as a member of a deliberative group
- Ability to read, understand, and interpret the organization's basic financial and operating statements

Special Competencies

(The number or percentage of board members who must possess each competency should be specified.)

(Continued)

Box 7.2. Continued

- Past experience serving on the board of other large or complex organizations or health care provider or financing organizations
- Experience as a senior health care executive
- Clinical experience (in medicine, nursing, or other allied field)
- Possession of specific expertise (such as managed care, corporate finance, law, information systems, labor relations, continuous quality improvement, mergers and acquisitions, organizational reengineering, or downsizing)

criteria to construct a profile of your board, a description of its present composition

2. Use the same set of criteria employed in step 1 to craft a profile of your board's ideal composition
3. Compare the actual and ideal profiles to develop a listing of specific member characteristics, capacities, and competencies your board needs in the future
4. Employ the listing developed in step 3 to identify, screen, and select new board members

PRINCIPLE 54

New board members participate in a carefully crafted and executed orientation process.

If the criteria-based profiling system we have described is employed, new members arrive at the boardroom door with the "right stuff," eager to make a contribution. However, a poor orientation process will impair their performance over the long run. Unfortunately, most board members are oriented (if at all) in a single, brief meeting with the CEO or board chair (see Box 7.3).

Figure 7.1. The Board Profiling Process

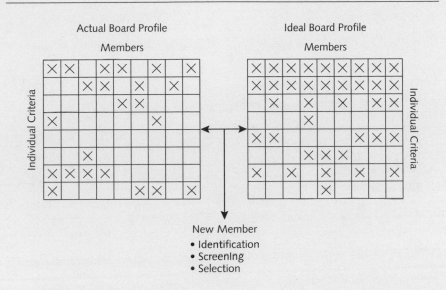

A truly effective new-member orientation process has the following characteristics:

- Someone (CEO, board chair, a senior board member) is assigned explicit responsibility for managing and overseeing the process.
- It is designed to accomplish specific objectives, such as

    Developing the basic knowledge and skills required to get started (not everything one must know to become a great board member)

    Introducing members to the climate and culture of the organization and board

    Helping new members feel a part of the group

    Motivating new members to begin participating and contributing

- It is a process, not a onetime event. We recommend that orientation take place throughout the new member's first year of service.
- Multiple approaches are employed, including

    One-on-one discussions and meetings (with the CEO, key executives, board chair, board standing committee chairs)

Tours of facilities

Organization-specific written materials

Books and articles

In-service programs and briefings

Attendance at extramural governance education programs

- Key subject matter is covered, including

Nature of the organization's environment (industry and market)

Characteristics of the most important stakeholder groups

The organization's vision, mission, and goals

Characteristics of the organization itself—its facilities, structure, management, services, programs, core competencies, competitors, challenges, and relationships with other organizations (suppliers, partners)

Characteristics of the physicians, clinical practice, and medical staff organization

An introduction to the board—its members, standing committees, mode of operation, culture, bylaws, objectives, policies, and work plans

The nature of governance obligations, responsibilities, roles, and duties

- It incorporates mentoring, whereby the new member is paired with an experienced, high-performing member of longer standing. The mentor's role is to serve as a guide, adviser, and counselor during the new member's first year. This is one of the most high-leverage orientation strategies.
- The process is periodically assessed and, if necessary, redesigned.

New board members are a precious asset. They must start off on the "right foot" and be nurtured to achieve their full potential.

PRINCIPLE 55

The board specifies its expectations of members.

There's an adage that says, "You will not get what you do not expect." To be effective, your board must agree on and communicate its expectations, and members must understand what is expected of them. Your board cannot demand accountability without this.

Some governance consultants recommend drafting a board member job description. We do not, because they have a tendency to be wordy, abstract, and imprecise. Rather, we encourage boards to simply list their most important expectations of members in two areas:

- *Citizenship*—basic expectations that are associated with board membership per se
- *Performance*—expectations that must be fulfilled by members for the board to discharge its obligations and fulfill its responsibilities

Some examples are provided in Box 7.4.

Once formulated, a list of member expectations can be employed in several ways. First, it is an explicit reminder and reinforcer of members' duties. Second, it can be given to prospective members during the recruitment

Box 7.4. Illustrative Board Member Expectations

Citizenship

All members are expected to

- Attend 90 percent of regularly scheduled board meetings each year
- Attend 80 percent of the regularly scheduled meetings of committees on which they serve
- Attend the annual board retreat
- Fulfill their fiduciary duty of loyalty, putting the interests of stakeholders ahead of their own
- Maintain confidentiality regarding all matters that demand it
- Do nothing that would discredit the organization

Performance

All members are expected to

- Arrive at board and committee meetings on time and not leave early
- Serve as members of at least two standing committees
- Carefully review background materials contained in the "agenda book" and come to board and committee meetings prepared
- Actively participate (by sharing ideas, opinions, observations, perspectives, expertise, and experience) in board and committee meeting deliberations and discussions
- Listen to and respect the opinions and perspectives of all other members
- Be willing to express a dissenting opinion and vote no when the need arises
- Fully support the board's policies and decisions once they have been implemented
- Serve as advocates of the organization in their dealings with other organizations, groups, and individuals

and selection process to answer the question the best candidates always ask: "What is expected of me if I were to join this board?" Third, it can serve as a set of criteria for periodically assessing the performance of individual members (addressed in Principle 57 later in this chapter).

PRINCIPLE 56

The board has fixed term lengths and limits the number of terms members can serve.

Term length is the number of years a board member serves before he or she must be renominated and reappointed. Term limits are the number of successive terms a member can serve before he or she must leave the board.

The rationale for term lengths is obvious. Without them, members would essentially hold their board seats in perpetuity. For this reason, most boards have set terms; two or three years is common.

The issue of term limits is more complex and hotly debated.

The case against them is based on the argument that performance and contribution need not necessarily decline with length of service. Indeed, experience is valuable. Boards benefit from having highly seasoned members. Furthermore, term limits are totally arbitrary and can result in the loss of talented and dedicated members.

We agree—*but* even the best boards generally find it difficult, if not impossible, not to invite members back at the conclusion of their term. To do otherwise is perceived as a public firing, which depreciates the member's past service, contributions, and self-worth. If boards had meaningful profiling (see Principle 53) and member assessment (see Principle 57) systems in place and if term renewal was not automatic but rather based on member performance and contributions in addition to organizational and board needs, term limits would be unnecessary. But that is typically not the case.

Therefore, as a practical measure, we recommend that your board institute term limits. It is the single best "fail-safe mechanism" for ensuring that your board's composition is continuously rejuvenated. We recommend three-year terms with a limit of three terms served. After a maximum of nine years, a member would be required to step down for a minimum of one year before he or she could be renominated. Under this arrangement, a board member has adequate time to learn the role, make a contribution, and assume a leadership position if so desired, yet it is short enough to guard against member burnout and board stagnation. The only exception should be an extension of no more than one term (or a portion thereof), if necessary, to assume or complete a term as board chair.

PRINCIPLE 57

The board periodically assesses the performance and contributions of every member; the results are employed to coach and develop members and make reappointment decisions.

Great boards are characterized by a culture of performance and accountability, not personality. Essential elements for building and maintaining this type of board are member assessment; feedback and member coaching as part of an individual development plan; and the absence of term renewal guarantees.

Individual member assessment is the "third rail" of governance; everyone recognizes its importance, but nobody wants to touch it. We estimate that fewer than 10 percent of health care organization boards have such a process in place. To effectively manage its composition, your board must assess the performance and contributions of individual members. This should be done for every board member prior to the conclusion of his or her term (before a decision is made whether to renominate) and should be based on explicit criteria drawn from your board's specification of member expectations (see Principle 55). Two different methodologies can be employed:

- *Self-assessment*—responding to a set of questions, the board member reflects on and assesses his or her own performance and contributions during the previous term.
- *360-degree assessment*—employing a standardized questionnaire, the board member is evaluated by each of his or her colleagues.

If your board does not have experience in this area, we recommend beginning with self-assessment; it is not threatening and is reasonably easy to undertake. Box 7.5 lists some questions that might be employed.

Undertaking a 360-degree assessment typically requires outside assistance to design a valid instrument and analyze the data. In addition, it often causes trepidation on the part of board members, both those being assessed and those doing the assessing. For these reasons, we recommend that it be used only after your board has become comfortable with self-assessment and skilled at employing it.

Box 7.5. Sample Board Member Self-Assessment Questions

- Do you continue to have the time, energy, and commitment to serve as a productive member of this board? What has been your level of attendance and participation at board and committee meetings?
- Over the long run, there must be some balance between what you get by serving on this board and the time and energy you expend as a member. What are the most important benefits you derive from being a member of this board?
- Objectively and candidly, rate your own performance and contributions in comparison to other members—are you among the lower third, middle third, or upper third?
- What are your most pronounced strengths as a board member?
- What are your most glaring weaknesses?
- What have been your distinctive contributions to this board during your last term?
- Which board member do you respect the most? What is it about this person's performance and contribution that you admire?
- What are four or five specific things you must do to become a better member of this board?

Feedback is useful only if it is employed to improve performance. Irrespective of the method employed, the insights gained from the assessment must be discussed with the member and then used to formulate a plan for continued development. Candidly talking with board members about their performance and contributions and working with them to improve both requires some special skills. Ideally, this task should be performed by the board chair; however, if the chair is unwilling or unable, it could be done by another senior board member. For obvious reasons, this cannot and should not be a responsibility of the CEO.

Assessment is an effective board composition management tool only if it precipitates change: improvement in a member's performance and contribution or removal from the board. For removal to be an option, your board must have an explicit policy that reads something like this:

> The ability of our board to make a difference and add value ultimately depends on the dedication, effort, and competencies of individual members. Accordingly, member term renewal is neither automatic nor guaranteed. The decision will be made on a case-by-case basis after a thorough assessment of the member's performance and contribution, his or her commitment to correct any deficiencies, and board and organizational needs.

PRINCIPLE 58

Board composition is nonrepresentational.

Of course, boards represent; they do so by balancing and aligning the needs, interests, and expectations of various stakeholder groups. The key notion is "balancing and aligning." What board members must not and cannot do is serve as the representative of a particular interest group or narrow interest (see Box 7.6). One board member seeks to advance the interests of one group and argues on its behalf; other members do the same thing from equally narrow perspectives. Members become advocates, and the boardroom takes on the characteristics of a courtroom or legislature. Boards are torn apart and rendered ineffective when this occurs.

Box 7.6. Predict the Future of This Board

Say you are a member of a hospital board where some members see themselves as representatives of and advocates for special interests:

- Harry feels that it is his duty to represent the interest of employees.
- Sarah, the chief of the medical staff serving on the board ex officio, sees herself as the advocate for physician interests (particularly those important to her specialty and the medical group in which she is a partner).
- Dan, the only black on the board, perceives himself as a representative of the African American community.
- Ann is the standard-bearer for women's issues and rights.
- Stephanie believes that as a nonprofit obligated to enhance community benefit, the hospital must cut costs to the bone; she views and assesses every issue from this perspective.
- John, who several years ago made the single largest gift the hospital has ever received, is concerned only about assuring his own legacy.

You predict: Would this board be able to govern on behalf of all stakeholders, or would it be torn apart and eventually rendered impotent by divergent array of very narrow interests and perspectives?

Representational governance can take on another face: the belief that a board's composition should mirror the characteristics of the stakeholder groups or community served—for example, 50 percent of the board should be women, 12 percent black, 8 percent Latino, so many from the bottom (or top) economic quartile, so many professionals, so many blue-collar workers, all living and working in the community, and so on. This approach is problematic for several reasons: First, given the size of most health care organization boards (fewer than twenty members) and the large number of social, demographic, ethnic, and economic attributes that would need to be "represented," it is impossible to achieve. Second, the primary characteristic of board members must be the willingness and ability to govern *on behalf of* all stakeholders and the community, not to match their collective profile of characteristics.

Don't misinterpret the preceding paragraph as an argument against diversity. Breadth of background, experience, and perspective is exceedingly valuable; it's the best safeguard against insular thinking and inappropriate pursuit of the status quo. Many boards are too white, too male, too middle-aged, too this, too that, and ultimately too narrow in their patterns of thinking; they lack the creativity that often comes with diversity to thrive in the midst of revolutionary change sweeping the health care industry.

PRINCIPLE 59

The CEO is a voting ex officio member of the board.

Ex officio members arrive at the boardroom door by virtue of another position they hold; they may be either voting or nonvoting. Such members might be executives of the organization, medical staff leaders, elected government officials, or officers of volunteer groups, to mention only several examples. In line with Principle 58, ex officio members, even though they come from a particular group, have the same obligations as any other board member: representing and balancing the interests of *all* stakeholders.

As previously addressed in Principles 13 through 20 in Chapter Four, the relationship between the CEO and your board is singularly important to the organization's success. This relationship has two facets: superior-subordinate and partner. The superior-subordinate aspect is reflected in the employment relationship. The board hires, guides and directs, determines the compensation of, and (when the need arises) fires the CEO. The partnership aspect of the relationship is made real and manifested by the CEO's voting board membership. The CEO's obligation to act on behalf of all stakeholders in addition to sharing responsibility and authority with the board is reinforced. The CEO is provided with "voice" inside the boardroom equal to that of the other members.

PRINCIPLE 60

In health care provider organizations, physicians should hold a significant number of board seats.

It is impossible to imagine an effective health care provider organization (such as a hospital) board that has no physician members. Clinical knowledge, experience, and perspective are needed in the boardroom. We are uncomfortable recommending a precise target, since circumstances and needs vary, but in most instances, 15 to 20 percent of board seats should be held by physicians. That is a large enough number to provide a diversity of clinical perspectives, yet small enough that physicians do not exercise disproportionate influence.

Physicians can be appointed ex officio (because of a medical staff leadership position they hold) or regularly elected. We recommend that only the chief or president of the medical staff be appointed ex officio and that other physicians be elected to the board through the same process as other members. Having all physician members appointed ex officio shifts critical composition management decisions from your board to the medical staff.

Regardless of the manner of appointment, physician members (in line with Principle 58) must balance and align the needs of all stakeholders; this fiduciary duty is breached if they represent just medical staff interests.

PRINCIPLE 61

"Insiders" and ex officio members make up less than 25 percent of the board's membership.

Inside board members (ex officio or not) are employees of the organization or individuals whose livelihood depends on it (members of the medical staff being the most common example).

After a period of time, insiders, no matter how well intentioned or high-minded, come to think of the organization as either an end in and of itself or a means to achieve their own professional aspirations. In both cases, their focus becomes directed inward: on the organization, its success, its growth, its survival. Your board's obligation is to ensure that the organization is a vehicle for advancing stakeholder interests. This critical focus can be compromised as the number of insiders increase.

Furthermore, as the number of ex officio members (whether insiders or outsiders) increase, the board begins to lose control of its own composition. Membership is determined by decisions made in the past (regarding the type of ex officio seats), and the locus of control shifts outside the board itself.

Although the maximum of 25 percent insiders and ex officio members is arbitrary, it does strike a balance between a board's need for the expertise insiders and ex officio members can bring to the board—the obligation of the board to be focused on stakeholders and the need for a board to control its own composition.

PRINCIPLE 62

Periodically, the board considers whether members should be compensated.

Whereas nearly 100 percent of commercial corporation boards compensate their members, only around 20 percent of nonprofit health systems and roughly 10 percent of nonprofit hospitals do. Board member compensation is a controversial issue that prompts passionate debate. Everyone seems to have a strongly held opinion, and it is split. We estimate that two-thirds of health care organization board members and CEOs think it is a bad idea; the other third feel it warrants serious consideration. A summary of the pros and cons is presented in Box 7.7.

To pay or not to pay? We do not have a recommendation, as the most important contextual considerations, constraints, sensitivities, and resulting costs and benefits are institutionally idiosyncratic. However, this is an important decision that should be made by design rather than by default (after careful board deliberation and debate) and then revisited every several years.

If your board decides to compensate members, here are some questions that should be addressed, along with our recommendations.

Box 7.7. To Compensate or Not to Compensate

The Cons

- Compensation of board members reinforces the increasingly prevalent notion that nonprofit health care organizations are no different from commercial enterprises and should be treated similarly in matters such as taxing revenues and property.
- The amount that most health care organizations are willing to pay board members would not make an appreciable difference in attracting or retaining the most able individuals, increasing meeting attendance, and stimulating participation.
- The compensation of nonprofit organization (particularly hospital) board members is an uncommon practice. Compensating boards members calls attention to the organization and demands justifications that may be misunderstood or misinterpreted.
- Board compensation is ill-timed given layoffs, marginal pay increases for employees, and other cost reduction efforts being initiated by many health systems and hospitals.
- Most present and prospective health care organization board members consider board service a civic responsibility; therefore, they neither want nor expect to be compensated. Paid service might offend the very individuals whom the organization most wants to attract and retain.
- When serving as organizational representatives or advocates, compensation might compromise board members' credibility. Their message might be perceived to have an implied disclaimer: "This is a paid endorsement."
- In some states, nonprofit organization board members are partially protected from personal liability, but only if they are unpaid. Compensation would jeopardize this indemnification.

(Continued)

Box 7.7. Continued

The Pros

- Board members expend a large amount of time, energy, and effort in performing their roles; they add significant value. Compensation is a tangible way for health care organizations to recognize and reward these valuable contributions.

- Board members incur both opportunity and indirect costs associated with their service. Compensation is a means to cover or reimburse these costs.

- The level of responsibility and accountability associated with serving on a health care organization board far exceeds that associated with other nonprofit organizations.

- Compensation makes it easier to attract and retain the most qualified and able individuals.

- Compensation stimulates better attendance and higher levels of participation at board and committee meetings.

- Compensation makes it easier to have higher expectations of board members and place greater demands on them.

- Commercial corporations compensate directors. Health care organization board membership is equally important and demanding. Therefore, such service warrants compensation.

- Compensation reinforces and increases board member accountability.

- Board members are typically successful individuals who, because of their involvement in a wide variety of business and community activities, have many demands placed on them. Compensation focuses member attention on their governance obligations and responsibilities.

- Compensation (particularly when it is significant) forces boards to get serious about new-member recruitment and selection and member evaluation. "Is this individual worth it?" then becomes a question that must be periodically confronted.

- Health care organizations are corporations valued in the hundreds of millions or even billions of dollars; they can afford to compensate board members.

- The behavior of many health systems and hospitals is indistinguishable from that of commercial corporations. Accordingly, there should be no differences in whether they compensate their board members or how much board members are paid.

- In general, you get what you pay for.

- What are the objectives of the program? What specific benefits will flow to stakeholders and the organization?

The only legitimate rationale for compensation is that it will enhance board performance and contributions and add stakeholder value. Objectives and benefits include the following:

Making it easier to attract and retain exceptionally well qualified and talented individuals

Encouraging more time and effort to be expended by board members

Increasing meeting attendance and participation

Reimbursing members for opportunity costs they inevitably incur in the course of board service

Reinforcing the importance of the work board members perform

- How should compensation be structured?

The options are a yearly retainer or a fee per board or committee meeting (or some combination of the two). A yearly retainer and a board (but not committee) meeting fee is the most effective and most justifiable arrangement. The retainer reinforces the importance or seriousness of the role in addition to rewarding talented and in-demand individuals for serving on the board. The per-meeting fee directly compensates members for their time.

- Should board members be actively discouraged from refusing compensation or donating their fees back to the organization?

If members are encouraged to "donate back" fees, the potential benefits that accrue to the organization from compensation are not realized.

- Should the board chair receive compensation in addition to that provided other members?

We say yes. The board chair is in a crucial leadership role that, if performed well, requires considerable time and energy. In many instances, compensation makes it a bit easier for busy and talented people to accept when asked to serve.

- Should some or all committee chairs receive a compensation differential?

For the sake of simplicity, we recommend not compensating committee chairs. If they are paid, a host of subsequent tricky questions arise, for example: Should all chairs be compensated? Should all chairs receive the same amount? When ad hoc committees are created, should their chairs be paid?

- Which board members, if any, should not be compensated?

Most plans exclude executives (such as the CEO) who serve on the board ex officio. Questions arise regarding whether medical staff officers (who are typically paid) should be separately compensated for board service; we recommend doing so.

- What should be the amount of compensation?

Many boards that decide to pay members make the mistake of setting the amount far below what is needed to accomplish their objectives. Our recommendation is that if a decision is made to compensate, do so at a level that grabs and focuses the attention of board members.

When fees are low, you will bear all of the negatives of compensation but gain few of the benefits.

- How should the compensation program be assessed to determine if stated objectives are being achieved?

A formal assessment of the extent to which the program meets its objectives, enhances board performance and contributions, and benefits stakeholders should be undertaken every several years.

- How, and how often, should fees be adjusted?

We recommend that the executive committee conduct a review every two years and make a recommendation to your board.

- How should the compensation program be explained or justified to key stakeholders, employees, the medical staff, and the community?

A specific, straightforward, and nondefensive rationale focusing on how the program benefits the organization and serves the interests of stakeholders should be developed prior to announcing the program.

CHECKUP

Composition

Respond to all questions.

	No	Not Entirely	Yes
1. My board proactively and consciously designs and manages its own composition.	1	2	3
2. New members of my board are recruited and selected on the basis of explicit criteria and as part of a profiling process.	1	2	3
3. New members of my board participate in a carefully crafted and executed orientation process.	1	2	3

	No	Not Entirely	Yes
4. My board specifies member expectations.	1	2	3
5. My board has fixed term lengths and limits the number of terms members can serve.	1	2	3
6. My board periodically assesses the performance of every member and employs the results to coach and develop them and make composition redesign decisions.	1	2	3
7. The composition of my board is "nonrepresentational"; members do not represent narrow constituencies or interest groups.	1	2	3
8. The CEO is a voting ex officio member of my board.	1		3
9. An appropriate number of physicians are members of my board.	1	2	3
10. Less than 25 percent of my board consists of insiders and ex officio members.	1	2	3
11. Every several years, my board considers whether board members should be compensated and if so, the method that will be employed to do so.	1	2	3

Total your responses for the eleven items, divide by 33, and then multiply by 100. The product is your board's percentage of the maximum score in this area.

Total _____ ÷ 33 × 100 = _____ percent

GETTING STARTED

✓ At an upcoming meeting, conduct a discussion of how, and how well, your board manages its composition. You might want to address some of the questions presented in Boxes 7.1 and 7.3.

✓ Develop a set of new board member selection criteria: basic qualifications, demographic characteristics, general competencies, and special competencies.

✓ Assign a committee the task of assessing, specifying the objectives for, and then designing a new-board-member orientation process.

✓ Devote some time at an upcoming meeting to identifying your board's most important expectations of members.

✓ If your board does not have fixed term lengths and limitations on the number of terms that can be served, debate the pros and cons of implementing them.

✓ If your board does not periodically assess the performance and contributions of individual members, design and implement a simple process for doing so. Consider using the questions in Box 7.5 to construct a member self-assessment.

✓ What proportion of your board is made up of insiders and ex officio members? How does it stack up against the 25 percent target figure recommended in Principle 61? Do such members represent and balance the interest of all stakeholders, or do they serve as advocates for narrow constituencies and interest groups?

✓ If the CEO is not a voting member of your board, spend some time at an upcoming meeting debating the pros and cons of changing that.

✓ Has your board recently considered whether members should be compensated? Using the pros and cons outlined in Box 7.7 as a starting point, analyze, discuss, and debate the potential assets and liabilities of doing so. The long and strong tradition of not paying members of health care organization boards can often put the brakes on a healthy discussion of this issue.

CHAPTER 8

Infrastructure

Boards are one of a health care organization's most important components, but typically, they are the least "well endowed" in terms of the infrastructure put in place to support them. Management and the medical staff require the right amount and mix of resources; so do boards.

Board infrastructure consists of the resources and systems necessary for facilitating the performance of governance work. The right infrastructure is essential because it increases the effectiveness and efficiency of a board's most valuable and scarcest assets, its own attention, time, and effort.

PRINCIPLE 63

The board has its own budget.

Few boards have their own budget, but having one is an excellent practice, for several reasons. First, your board should subject itself to the same financial discipline it expects of the organization as a whole. Second, budgeting gives your board an opportunity to plan for the resources it needs. Third, having a budget eliminates the necessity of requesting funds from management on an ad hoc, item-by-item basis. Fourth, an annual budget is the best way to account for the true costs of governance.

At the beginning of each fiscal year, the executive committee, led by the board chair, should prepare a draft budget, which is then discussed and approved by the board. Several categories of expenditures should be included:

- *Staffing*—proportions of salaries and benefits for personnel who provide staff and secretarial support to the board
- *Services*—board consultation, governance-specific legal assistance, directors' and officers' liability insurance
- *Operations*—supplies, telephone, duplication and printing, postage and mailing, food service (at meetings), reimbursed member meeting attendance expenses, board member compensation (if any)
- *Education and development*—materials, books, subscriptions, memberships, member participation in educational conferences, fees and expenses associated with conducting periodic board retreats

PRINCIPLE 64

The board has adequate staff support.

The proper amount and type of staff support is a crucial element of infrastructure. Most boards are staffed, as one of many duties, by the CEO's assistant or secretary, typically one of the most overloaded and overworked employees in the organization. As a consequence, board support can get squeezed or moved to a back burner. A person (senior executive assistant or secretary) should be assigned the function of "board coordinator," assuming responsibility for both providing and directing governance staff support. A specific proportion of the person's time should be allocated to this role and reflected in your board's budget. In addition, the board coordinator's functions should be specified in an explicit job description (see Box 8.1 for an example).

PRINCIPLE 65

The board formulates annual governance objectives.

The development of annual objectives is a great tool for planning, focusing, and organizing your board's work.

At the beginning of each year, the executive committee should specify the most important things your board must accomplish. The committee's

Box 8.1. Sample Board Coordinator Position Description

The board requires excellent staff support to optimize its performance. An individual will be assigned the function of *board coordinator.*

Position

The person performing this function is _____, presently occupying the position of _____. It is estimated that _____ percent of his/her time will be devoted to governance staffing. For administrative purposes, this person reports to the CEO; in fulfilling the tasks described below, the board coordinator works with, and is accountable to, the CEO and board chair.

Key Tasks

- Planning for, coordinating, and managing other support staff who work with the board and its committees
- Preparing agendas and supporting materials for board and committee meetings
- Compiling and distributing materials ("agenda books") for all board and committee meetings
- Recording policies and decisions at board and committee meetings
- Maintaining all board records
- Maintaining a file of board policies and decisions
- Ensuring that analyses, reports, and other materials requested by the board are prepared
- Serving as the point of first contact for board member requests
- Making preparations for board educational sessions and retreats
- Handling all board-related correspondence
- Performing other duties as requested by the CEO, the chair, and their designees to support effective and efficient board functioning

draft objectives should then be discussed, modified if necessary, and then approved by your board. The question is, what are the most important things your board must achieve in order to meet its obligations and fulfill its responsibilities? Sample board's governance objectives are presented in Box 8.2.

Carefully conceived, explicit and precise governance objectives, formulated annually, provide the basis for

- Crafting agendas and managing meetings (Principles 66 and 67)
- Developing committee charges and work plans (Principle 50)
- Designing education and development activities (Principles 70 and 71)
- Board assessment (Principle 72)

Box 8.2. Sample Governance Objectives

- Develop and implement a plan to increase board members' involvement in key community groups and improve their input to our governance process.

- Identify key organizational stakeholders and begin the process of understanding what they want from and expect of the organization.

- Review and, if necessary, redraft the organization's vision statement, increasing its specificity regarding core purposes and values.

- Explore the benefits and feasibility of merging with a regionally based health care delivery system.

- Develop a CEO succession plan.

- Retain a consultant to conduct an audit (of characteristics, of strengths and weaknesses) of the medical credentialing process.

- Have at least five members of the board, accompanied by the CEO, participate in the XYZ Governance Conference.

- Develop charters and annual objectives for all board standing committees.

144

PRINCIPLE 66

Meeting agendas are carefully devised plans for deploying the board's attention and time.

Legally and functionally, your board exists only when it meets—"between raps of the gavel." Board meetings are the epicenter of governance; they are where the work gets done. The way meetings are planned and conducted, in addition to the dynamics that emerge in them, significantly affects governance quality. Meetings must effectively and efficiently deploy your board's time and focus member attention on the most important issues.

Board agendas are often little more than a listing of topics put together at the last moment with minimal forethought. When this is the case, they cannot provide the foundation for productive and creative board meetings.

Most agenda items come from four sources: proposed by management, forwarded by the medical staff, based on your board's annual objectives, or resulting from board committee work. The executive committee should convene (either face to face or by teleconference) several weeks prior to each board meeting to set the agenda based on these inputs, deciding which items should be scheduled and for each, the objective sought, how much time should be allocated, and the type of background material needed to prepare board members to address it.

Your board must have a plan or a budget for allocating its meeting time; our recommendations appear in Box 8.3.

Here are some agenda planning and management tips:

- Meetings should not be held concurrently with meals. Doing so wastes time and deflects attention. "Breaking bread" can be a very useful communal experience and catalyst, but such activities should occur before or after meetings or be separately scheduled.
- Without exception, meetings should begin and conclude on time. The starting and ending times noted on the agenda should never be compromised. This conveys an attitude of seriousness and efficiency, in addition to respecting the value of members' time.

Box 8.3. A Board Meeting Agenda

AGENDA

MEETING OF THE BOARD

Place: Conference Room A

Date: Wednesday, March 13, 2002

Start time: 5:00 P.M.

End time: 8:30 P.M.

Important: Please confirm your attendance by calling Ms. Howell at 123-4567.

General

1. Reflection: role of the board as a representative for and advocate of the disadvantaged and underserved in our service area *(Presenter: Ms. Hammel, chair)*

    Time allocated: 5:00 P.M. to 5:10 P.M.

    Background: Executive summary of community health status and needs assessment survey; agenda book, Tab A

2. Approvals *(Ms. Hammel)*:

    Board meeting minutes of 2/11/02

    Designated Medicaid provider certification

    Joint Commission final report (previously discussed in draft form at meeting of 1/12/02)

    Board employee service award recognitions

    Objective: Consent

    Time allocated: 5:10 P.M. to 5:15 P.M.

    Background: Agenda book, Tab B

Ends

3. Charity care *(Mr. Jacobs, chair, Vision and Goals Committee)*
   Objective: Policy formulation
   Time allocated: 5:15 P.M. to 5:30 P.M.
   Background: Draft policy alternatives and recommendations;
   agenda book, Tab C

Executive Performance

4. CEO report *(Mr. Samuelson, president/CEO)*
   Objective: Information, Q&A
   Time allocated: 5:30 P.M. to 5:50 P.M.
   Background: Audio tape included with agenda book

5. Revised employment contract and severance agreement *(Mr. Benson,*
   Executive Performance and Compensation Committee)
   Objective: Decision
   Time allocated: 5:50 P.M. to 6:10 P.M.
   Background: Agenda book, Tab C

Quality

6. Medical staff credentialing *(Dr. Hauer, chair, Quality Committee)*
   Objective: Decisions
   Time allocated: 6:10 P.M. to 6:30 P.M.
   Background: Agenda book, Tab D

7. Revised quality indicators and standards *(Dr. Hauer)*
   Objective: Policy, oversight
   Time allocated: 6:30 P.M. to 6:50 P.M.
   Background: Agenda book, Tab E

(Continued)

Box 8.3 Continued

Finance

8. Auditor's report *(Mr. Williams, Collen, Powell & Hovell, CPAs)*

    Objective: Oversight

    Time allocated: 6:50 P.M. to 7:30 P.M.

    Background: Executive summary included in agenda book, Tab F; full report provided as separate attachment

9. Executive session with audit partner *(Ms. Hammel, Mr. Williams)*

    Objective: Oversight

    Time allocated: 7:30 P.M. to 8:00 P.M.

    Background: See item 8.

Governance

10. Nomination of Mr. Jacob Nester as a new member of the board *(Ms. Kraus, chair, Governance Committee)*

    Objective: Decision

    Time allocated: 8:00 P.M. to 8:15 P.M.

    Background: Résumé and committee assessment; agenda book, Tab G

11. Meeting assessment *(Ms. Hammel)*

    Objective: Oversight

    Time allotted: 8:15 P.M. to 8:30 P.M.

    Background: None

Note: After the meeting, a cocktail reception and dinner will be hosted at Cajun Joe's Restaurant to welcome Mr. Jon Andrews, the hospital's newly appointed chief operating officer. Confirm your attendance by calling Ms. Howell at 123-4567. Please make every effort to join us.

- In all but the most unusual circumstances, board meetings should not be scheduled to last more than three hours. Attention and energy generally begin to wane after this period of time.

- Most boards make the mistake of overestimating the number of items that can be thoughtfully discussed, deliberated, and acted on. Recall how many times in the past several years your board did not get through the agenda or had to meet longer than planned. Less is generally better; place fewer, rather than more, items on the agenda.

- In considering potential agenda items, the executive committee should ask: Why should your board be dealing with this issue? Is it critical to fulfilling its obligation and responsibilities? Is this a matter on which your board must "weigh in" and can add substantial value? A proposed item should be rejected unless the strongest case can be made for including it.

- For each agenda item, the type of issue and its objective should be noted. Issues coming before your board require policy formulation, decision making, or oversight regarding ends, executive performance, quality, finances, or your board's own effectiveness and efficiency. Classifying each agenda item by both responsibility and role reinforces the fundamental (and most important) aspect of your board's work. Furthermore, each item should have an explicit objective. There are four possibilities:

  Consent items are routine "housekeeping" matters that do not warrant discussion and deliberation but require board approval. They are grouped as a single agenda item. Members review these materials prior to the meeting, and if no one has any questions or concerns, the entire block is acted on with a single vote and no discussion. This can free up a significant amount of time that might otherwise be squandered on minor issues. Any member can request that an individual item be discussed and voted on separately.

  Information items are points that should be made but for which no discussion or action is necessary; questions and requests for clarification are entertained.

Discussion items are matters the board talks about and provides input on, an exchange takes place, but no action is necessary.

Action items are the meeting's main business. These are issues requiring discussion, deliberation, and a vote—policies, decisions, and matters requiring oversight.

• A precise amount of time should be allocated to each item. Again, it pays to be a bit liberal here; overestimating the time needed to address an issue causes fewer problems that underestimating. If more time is needed to handle an item, a decision should be made on the spot by the chair regarding which items will receive less time or be tabled. This process, when employed consistently, disciplines your board in setting priorities and using its time efficiently.

• Each item should have an individual assigned to make a presentation (if needed), answer questions, and facilitate the discussion.

• Resource materials supporting each item should be prepared and included in the agenda book. Include only materials that are absolutely necessary to help members understand an issue, ask questions, and engage in a thoughtful discussion. Agenda books should be distributed to board members about a week preceding the meeting; this provides enough time for review but is not so far in advance that the agenda is relegated to the bottom of people's "to do" pile.

• The same agenda planning and management system should be employed by all of your board's committees.

PRINCIPLE 67

Board meetings are managed and conducted in a way that promotes high levels of effectiveness, efficiency, and creativity.

We've all experienced them far too often: mind-numbing, deenergizing, unfocused meetings that accomplish little and waste members' time. Whether your board meetings are productive depends, in addition to

Getting to Great

agenda planning, on how well they are managed and facilitated. Here are a few recommendations.

Begin with some type of brief activity that reinforces your board's obligation and responsibilities. One of the best illustrations of this practice we've seen occurred on a Catholic hospital board on which one of us sat. The chair started each meeting by making an observation or posing a question dealing with some "big picture" aspect of governance, typically related to an important agenda item. She would then ask members to share their reflections. The board looked forward to these discussions. They helped members transcend the detail and focus attention on the board's purpose and what must be done to achieve it.

Never back up and summarize what has transpired for members arriving late. This wastes the time of those who were prompt.

The broader aspects of board leadership will be the focus of Principle 68. However, first and foremost, the chair must either possess or be willing to quickly acquire the knowledge and skills necessary to run productive meetings. Since chair facilitation skills significantly influence meeting effectiveness, efficiency, and creativity, incumbents should be required to develop them. Various resources are available for doing so:

- Continuing education programs and workshops offered by local colleges and professional or trade associations
- A number of excellent books on the subject (see Box 8.4)
- Tutoring by board members, staff, or other individuals who have well-developed skills in this area

Every effort should be made to maximize the amount of meeting time members spend interacting rather than passively listening (consider the questions posed in Box 8.5); talk is the way your board's work gets accomplished. Far too much precious meeting time is spent conveying information that can be better presented in other ways, for example:

- Include in the agenda book a summary of key information needed to understand an issue.

Box 8.4. Resources to Help You Run Better Meetings

- *Meetings That Work! A Practical Guide to Shorter and More Productive Meetings,* by Richard Y. Chang and Kevin R. Kehoe (San Francisco: Jossey-Bass/Pfeiffer, 1999)

- *First Aid for Meetings,* by Charlie Hawkins (Wilsonville, Ore.: Book Partners, 1997)

- *The Strategy of Meetings,* by George David Kieffer (New York: Warner Books, 1988)

- *How to Run a Successful Meeting—in Half the Time,* by Milo O. Frank (New York: Simon & Schuster, 1989)

- *How to Make Meetings Work! The New Interaction Method,* by Michael Doyle and David Straus (New York: Berkley, 1993)

Box 8.5. Listening and Talking

How much of your board meeting time is spent passively listening (to presentations of background materials, briefings, committee reports, and so on)? How much is spent actively interacting, with members discussing, questioning, deliberating, and weighing alternatives? The ratio for most boards is about 60 percent to 40 percent. Although clearly extreme, consider a board that spends all of its time—every moment of every meeting—just listening. Could it really govern? Obviously not. There would be no discussion, no questions, no deliberation, no weighing of alternatives, no interchange of ideas, no debate; all of which are necessary for acting—for formulating policy, making decisions, and overseeing.

- Some briefing materials cannot be effectively and efficiently conveyed in writing (or it just takes too much effort to prepare). When greater richness is required, consider making a brief audiotape to supplement written materials and include it with the agenda package.

Do not spend meeting time re-presenting or even summarizing information previously provided in the agenda book; expect and assume that it has been read and digested. Meeting time can then be spent responding to questions and discussion.

Often in handling specific agenda items, a board's process is haphazard; members are not in sync—an issue is presented, several members express their opinions, a few others ask for clarification regarding alternatives, someone else questions whether the board should even be dealing with the matter at all, and so on. To be effective, your board must focus its attention and be together in doing so. In considering a given agenda item, we recommend the following steps that members move through in sequence, together:

1. Fully understand the matter at hand and define it precisely.

2. Clarify assumptions.

3. Specify alternative solutions or choices.

4. Weigh and assess alternatives.

5. Resolve the issue: make your choice, formulate the policy, or reach a decision.

6. Determine the follow-up activities required, if any.

If your board conducts its meetings using *Robert's Rules of Order,* consider not doing so. First developed in the 1800s, these practices were designed to manage deliberation and decision making by very large legislative bodies. This highly structured and rigid process is inappropriate and unnecessarily cumbersome for small groups such as boards. It can sap creativity and impede, rather than facilitate, meeting effectiveness and efficiency.

Most board minutes resemble a transcript, attempting to capture the flow of discussion taking place in a meeting. Compiled in this way, they require huge amounts of effort to produce and result in documents that are largely symbolic and have little substantive value. Rather than taking traditional minutes, consider using a form such as the one in Figure 8.1 to summarize each agenda item. In addition to noting the type of item and objective, key discussion points are summarized as a brief bulleted list, background materials included in the agenda book are noted, and the follow-up required is specified. Attached to the form, where appropriate, is the policy or decision summary form (see Chapter Five and Figures 5.2 and 5.3).

Allocate about ten minutes at the end of each meeting to evaluate how well your board planned for and used its time. Some questions that might be posed and discussed are presented in Box 8.6. At first, expect reticence; with time and persistence, the effort will bear fruit.

Box 8.6. Board Meeting Evaluation Questions

- Did the agenda book contain useful information in a form that helped members understand the issues? How could the materials be improved?

- Did members come to the meeting fully prepared?

- Did the agenda focus on important issues, those demanding board attention where real value can be added? What agenda items should have been eliminated? Which warranted more time?

- What proportion of the board meeting was spent talking versus listening? What can be done to increase the percentage?

- Did members have ample opportunity to ask questions and express their opinions?

- Was the meeting effective, efficient, and creative?

- What specific member behaviors were most helpful? What behaviors were counterproductive?

- How effective was the chair's facilitation of the meeting? What might he or she have done better or differently?

Figure 8.1. Form for Recording Board Meeting Minutes

Agenda Item Summary Form

Meeting date: _____

Item number: _____

Type: ☐ Consent

☐ Ends

☐ Executive performance

☐ Quality

☐ Finances

☐ Self

Objective: ☐ Information

☐ Discussion

☐ Action—policy

☐ Action—decision

☐ Action—oversight

Key discussion point summary:

Decision or policy summary form attached ☐

Background materials included in the agenda book:

Follow-up required:

PRINCIPLE 68

The chair is carefully selected, understands his or her role, and is able to perform it effectively.

A great chair does not guarantee high levels of board performance, but a poor one always seriously undermines it.

The board chair must be able to perform four roles:

- *A ceremonial and representational role*—symbolizing, representing, and being a spokesperson to internal and external constituents
- *A leadership role:*—influencing, motivating, organizing, focusing, and monitoring the board and the way it goes about its work
- *A facilitative role*—planning and conducting effective, efficient, and creative board meetings (addressed in Principle 67)
- *A consultative role*—serving as a confidant and adviser to the CEO on organizational and governance issues and executive-board relationships

The chair should be selected with great care, based on his or her ability to perform these roles. The position should not be a reward for long tenure or past contributions, nor should it be offered to a member because of his or her status or availability.

The term of the chair in most health care organizations is one year; we recommend two years. This provides an adequate amount of time to get comfortable with the role and then make a contribution.

Typically, the vice chair moves into the position of chair. Having served as vice chair provides the time and opportunity for an incumbent to develop the needed knowledge and skills. However, we feel it unwise for there to be a set sequence of positions for members automatically to move through on the way to becoming the chair (for example, treasurer to secretary to vice chair to chair). This practice locks a board into a succession arrangement in which the chair is actually selected many years in advance. Problems, opportunities, and board needs change; flexibility in selection of the chair is therefore a must.

Selection and execution of the chair's position should be guided by a job description, an illustration of which is provided in Box 8.7. Not only

Box 8.7. Board Chair Job Description

The board chair is a critical leadership position. How, and how well, the occupant performs this role has a significant impact on our board's performance and contribution.

The chairperson, working cooperatively with the CEO, leads the board. He or she serves as a representative to both internal and external constituencies and is an important member of the organization's leadership team.

Responsibilities

- Serves as a counselor and adviser to the CEO on governance and board-executive relations
- Serves as the board's representative to key stakeholder groups
- Facilitates board meetings, ensuring that they are focused, effective, efficient, and creative
- Serves as a mentor to other board members
- Serves as the board's contact with the media
- Chairs the board's executive committee
- With the advice and consent of the executive committee, designates the chairs of board committees
- Serves as an ex officio member of all board committees (but is not, except in the rarest instances, expected to participate in their work and deliberations)
- With assistance provided by the executive committee,
  Drafts the board's annual objectives
  Develops the board's work plan
  Formulates agendas for all board meetings
- Assumes other responsibilities and performs other tasks as directed by the board

(Continued)

Box 8.7. Continued

Qualifications

- Has determined, after careful self-assessment and reflection, that he or she has the time, energy, and desire to assume this demanding position
- Has at least four years of experience as a member of the board
- Has in-depth knowledge of the organization's challenges and opportunities, structure, functioning, and programs and services
- Thoroughly understands the governance process
- Has received an "outstanding" rating on all prior board member performance evaluations
- Has no conflicts of interest that would prohibit him or her from acting in the best interests of the organization and its stakeholders
- Is respected for his or her personal and professional integrity, wisdom, intelligence, and judgment by the board, the management team, and physician leaders
- Has a collegial working relationship with the CEO
- Has a collegial working relationship with other board members

Term

The tenure of the board chair shall be an uninterrupted two-year term. If an individual's term as chair should end beyond the maximum term limit for board members, that limit shall be extended to allow the individual to complete his or her term as chair.

Nominations and Election

Nominees for the position of chair need not have served as a board officer, but their having served at least one term on the board's executive committee is useful (though not mandatory). A special committee shall submit to the board one or more nominees for the position of chair. This committee shall be composed of the present board chair, the CEO, one at-large board member (elected by the full board), and one former chair not presently serving on the board (elected by the board).

does this provide a way to hold the chair accountable, but it also facilitates the individual's orientation, development, and evaluation.

PRINCIPLE 69

The CEO does not serve as the board's chair.

Combining the CEO and board chair roles is common in the commercial sector. Nevertheless, although the CEO should be a member of the board (see Principle 59), he or she should *not* be the chair, for two important reasons:

- When these important roles are combined, the already fuzzy line that differentiates management and governance work is further blurred. Confusion and conflict regarding authority and responsibilities often result.

- This dual role concentrates too much power in the hands of one person. The CEO, already possessing considerable influence due to his or her full-time presence, access to information, and control of the organization's resources, can totally dominate a board.

Boards serve to check and balance stakeholders' interests within the organization; the scale is tipped when the CEO is also the board's chair.

PRINCIPLE 70

The board is serious about continuous member development and has a plan for accomplishing it.

When entering the boardroom for the first time, no member possesses all of the knowledge and skills he or she will need; moreover, new issues emerge constantly, and both board needs and organizational challenges and opportunities change over time. Hence continuous member development is essential. And it begins with new-member orientation (see Principle 54).

The quality of board work is the result of, and is constrained by, its members' knowledge and skills. Your board must have a plan to enhance its capacities, supported by a budget for doing so (see Principle 63). Here are some key elements:

- Conduct periodic board retreats. This is so important that it is addressed separately (as Principle 71).

- Include several carefully selected articles on emerging trends and issues in each agenda book, and allocate a small amount of meeting time to discuss them. This practice reinforces the importance of continuous learning and provides an efficient way for pursuing it. Management staff, the chair, and board members should be on the lookout for suitable materials.

- Enter subscriptions for all board members to key magazines and newsletters dealing with both substantive (industry, market, organizational) and governance issues (for some recommendations, see Box 8.8).

- Several times each year, distribute a thoughtfully selected book on governance to board members (for some recommendations, see Box 8.9).

- Have management (with guidance and direction supplied by the chair) prepare briefing books on important issues and matters that will be coming before your board. This is one of the most effective development strategies because it is targeted; necessity always provides the most

---

Box 8.8. Governance Magazines and Newsletters

- *Trustee*—monthly magazine published by the American Hospital Association; (800) 621-6902

- *American Governance Leader*—monthly newsletter published by the American Governance and Leadership Group; (909) 336-1586

- *Health Governance Report*—monthly newsletter published by Opus Publications; (800) 650-6787

- *The Board Report*—free monthly newsletter published by Ernst & Young; (800) 726-7339

Box 8.9. Books on Governance

- *Board Work: Governing Health Care Organizations,* by Dennis D. Pointer and James E. Orlikoff (San Francisco: Jossey-Bass, 1999)

- *Boards That Make a Difference: A New Design for Leadership in Nonprofit and Public Organizations,* by John Carver (San Francisco: Jossey-Bass, 1997)

- *The Effective Board of Trustees,* by Richard P. Chait, Thomas P. Holland, and Barbara E. Taylor (Westport, Conn.: Oryx Press, 1993)

- *The Future of Health Care Governance: Redesigning Boards for a New Era,* by James E. Orlikoff and Mary K. Totten (Chicago: American Hospital Publishing, 1996)

- *Practical Governance,* by J. Larry Tyler and Errol Biggs (Chicago: Health Administration Press, 2001)

- *Really Governing: How Health Systems and Hospital Boards Can Make More of a Difference,* by Dennis D. Pointer and Charles M. Ewell (Albany, N.Y.: Delmar, 1994)

- *The Trustee Handbook for Health Care Governance,* by James E. Orlikoff and Mary K. Totten (San Francisco: Jossey-Bass, 2001)

powerful motivation to learn. For example, if a merger or acquisition is being considered, a briefing book might be prepared on your board's involvement in the due diligence process and its duties in reviewing and approving "big deals."

- On a rotating basis, small groups of members should be sent to governance-related conferences, seminars, and workshops. This practice gives members the opportunity to be exposed to a broad range of ideas and issues. Some suggestions are noted in Box 8.10.

PRINCIPLE 71

The board holds periodic retreats.

Retreats (people who object to the negative military connotation call them "advances") provide a unique opportunity for board education and discussion and a forum for addressing issues not possible at board meetings. Annual or semiannual retreats can help your board prepare for the future, grow, change, rejuvenate itself, and become more effective.

We facilitate more than eighty board retreats a year. Here are some recommendations, focusing on both context and substance, for designing and conducting great ones.

- Assign the responsibility for planning to your board's executive or governance committee. This should be an ongoing activity throughout the year, not something done at the last moment.

- Schedule the event far in advance; we recommend at least six months. This is the best way to ensure a high level of attendance. Little is gained by holding a retreat when only a portion of the board is present.

- Select a specific objective, theme, or issue that will serve as the retreat's focus. Make sure it is something that cannot be effectively addressed at regularly scheduled meetings. "Retreating" to conduct routine business is a waste of time and money. Most topics fall into the following categories:

General education and development

Reviewing and analyzing results of a board assessment and engaging in action planning to improve performance and contributions (see Principle 72)

Developing the annual board objectives and work plan

Board team building

Gaining a better understanding of industry or market trends, competitors, and partners

Building more effective relationships between the board and management

Addressing significant future organizational and board challenges and opportunities

- Make it a true retreat—a withdrawal from the harried day-to-day work environment to a less frantic and less distracting place where people can relax, focus their attention, and release their creativity. Seize the opportunity to "get out of town." The venue need not be far away or expensive.

- Take advantage of the chance for board, management, and physician leaders to interact in ways that might be difficult back home. Do everything you can to encourage and facilitate this. For example, make all meals communal events; this maximizes inclusion and interaction.

- Celebrate organizational and board accomplishments.

- Consider retaining the services of an experienced consultant to serve as a facilitator; make these arrangements well in advance. The best talent is in great demand. Facilitator quality, more than any other factor, will determine your retreat's success. Ask for references, and talk with several past clients. The most effective facilitators are "entertaining experts," combining broad, in-depth expertise and experience with the ability to convey ideas in an engaging, powerful, and stimulating way.

- Allocate at least 50 percent of the retreat meeting time to discussion. Just sitting and listening to speakers (no matter how talented) is deadly and squanders a tremendous opportunity for enlightened engagement around key issues.

- Include an action-planning component. The board must walk away with a precise notion of "what comes next."

- Work from a budget; retreats can be expensive.

- Formally evaluate all aspects of the retreat. Incorporate this evaluation into the planning for next year's event.

PRINCIPLE 72

The board engages in a periodic self-assessment and formulates action plans to improve its performance and contributions.

Assessment, feedback, analysis, and action planning are critical practices for continually enhancing governance quality. Individual board member assessment was addressed in Principle 57; we turn here to evaluating the board as a whole.

By design or by default, boards continually assess themselves. But unless these perceptions are systematically collected, organized, shared, analyzed, and acted on, they will not lead to better governance. Accordingly, your board should engage in a periodic (we recommend every other year) assessment of the things that most affect its performance and contributions:

- How well your board discharges its responsibility for ends, executive performance, quality, and finances

- The appropriateness of your board's structure, composition, and infrastructure

A questionnaire, self-designed or obtained from an outside source, should be employed to gather members' perceptions.

Recognize, however, that assessment per se, no matter how well done, never improves performance. The information collected must be fed back to and analyzed and discussed by your board. Using the results, your board must develop action plans for improving how it governs. We recommend that these activities take place at a special board meeting or retreat.

164

CHECKUP

Infrastructure

Respond to all items.

	No	Not Entirely	Yes
1. My board has its own budget.	1		3
2. My board has adequate staff support.	1	2	3
3. My board formulates annual governance objectives.	1	2	3
4. My board's meeting agendas are carefully planned.	1	2	3
5. My board's meetings are well managed and facilitated; they are effective, efficient, and creative.	1	2	3
6. The chair is carefully selected, understands his or her role, and is able to perform it effectively.	1	2	3
7. The chair of my board is the CEO.	3		1
8. My board is serious about continual member development and has a plan to accomplish it.	1	2	3
9. My board holds a retreat at least every other year.	1		3
10. My board periodically assesses its performance and contributions and, employing the results, engages in action planning to improve governance quality.	1	2	3

Total your responses for the ten items, divide by 30, and then multiply by 100. The product is your board's percentage of the maximum score in this area.

Total _____ ÷ 30 × 100 = _____ percent

GETTING STARTED

✓ Conduct an audit of your board's infrastructure.

How adequate is it?

Does your board have the appropriate mix of resources it needs to govern effectively and efficiently?

What is missing?

What elements of infrastructure must be put in place to optimize your board's performance and contributions?

✓ Allocate some time at an upcoming meeting to discuss and then "sketch out" about a half dozen of the most important objectives your board must accomplish over the next year. Develop some initial work plans.

✓ Have a frank discussion about the effectiveness, efficiency, and creativity of your board's meetings. What are the positives and negatives? Consider implementing some of the recommendations made in this chapter: agenda planning, agenda format, policy and decision-making summary forms, not using *Robert's Rules of Order,* and revising the minute-taking process.

✓ Analyze the quality of your board's leadership: the chair position in general and its present occupant. This is tough to do in a meeting. Therefore, we suggest that all members be asked to respond anonymously, in writing, to some questions, such as these:

What are the most pronounced strengths of the board chair?

What are the chair's greatest weaknesses (and developmental opportunities)?

What specific things should the chair do, stop doing, and do better to lead more effectively?

How could the position of board chair be strengthened?

The responses should be collated, organized, and discussed by the executive committee. Based on this, a list of leadership issues should be prepared and discussed with the chair, who should then develop a performance improvement action plan.

✓ At a meeting, pose the following questions:

How serious is our board about continual member development?

What important knowledge, skills, and perspectives are we lacking?

What initiatives should be mounted to develop our board's competencies and capacities?

✓ If your board does not undertake a periodic self-assessment or does it poorly, consider implementing or revising the process.

CHAPTER 9

Implementing Principle-Based Governance

Chapters Two through Eight have dealt with *what* your board must do to improve its performance and contribution; this chapter focuses on *how*. There are five components:

- Understanding the principles of great governance
- Assessing your board
- Formulating a set of principles, tailored to your board, specifying how it will govern
- Undertaking governance transformation work as a team
- Dealing with the challenges of mounting and sustaining significant change efforts

CHARACTERISTICS OF GREAT GOVERNANCE

Engineering change begins with a vivid, rich, and empowering image of what your board should be like at its very best. By reading this book, you are there. You understand the principles of health care organization governance—best practices regarding board obligations, responsibilities, roles, structure, composition, and infrastructure. They provide your board with a "magnetic north," the direction in which it should head.

ASSESSMENT

To begin moving toward a goal, one has to know where one is at present. By completing the Checkups in Chapters Two through Eight, you have done most of the work. What remains is bringing everything together and doing some analysis and reflection.

Step 1

Enter scores for each Checkup in the appropriate box.

Board basics (Chapter Two, page 14) _____
Obligations (Chapter Three, page 28) _____
Ends (Chapter Four, page 40) _____
Executive performance (Chapter Four, page 50) _____
Quality (Chapter Four, page 62) _____
Finances (Chapter Four, page 69) _____
Roles (Chapter Five, page 90) _____
Structure (Chapter Six, page 111) _____
Composition (Chapter Seven, page 137) _____
Infrastructure (Chapter Eight, page 165) _____
TOTAL _____

Divide the total by 10 to get your summary score:

SUMMARY SCORE _____ percent

Step 2

Plot each score by placing a dot on each of the appropriate axes in Figure 9.1. Then connect them to form a "spider diagram."

The *summary score* is an indicator of your board's overall fitness: above 80 percent is exemplary; between 60 and 80 percent is adequate; below 60 percent is problematic; impaired is under 40 percent.

The spider diagram in Figure 9.1 is a graphical profile of your board across the dimensions of governance that most affect its performance and contributions.

Figure 9.1. Your Board's Practice Profile

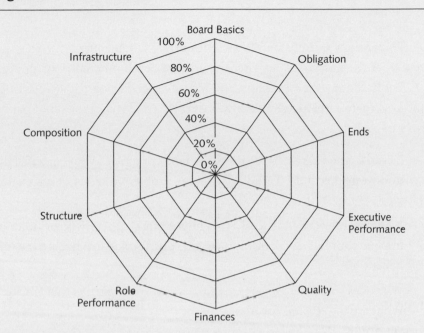

For dimensions rated above 80 percent, ask the following questions:

- Was your initial assessment candid and accurate? Look over the Checkups that resulted in high scores. Review each of the individual items and your responses to them. Most self-assessments suffer from a "halo effect." Step back and be really tough on your board. Change your ratings as necessary, and recompute the scores where appropriate.

- Which of your board's characteristics and practices are truly outstanding? To build high levels of spirit and motivation, your board must recognize what it does well. In addition, areas of high performance can deteriorate over time. What should your board be doing to celebrate, reinforce, and maintain excellence?

- Are there problem areas? Although your overall score on a particular dimension might be high, there may be Checkup items to which you gave low scores. Do not overlook them. These are weeds in a patch of roses.

Dimensions rated below 60 percent warrant careful attention. They are your board's weaknesses but offer the greatest development opportunities.

Look through the Checkups, and identify specific board characteristics and governance practices rated low. List each on a separate sheet of paper. For each:

- Describe the characteristic or governance practice. What, specifically, does your board do (or not do) that is problematic? Jot down examples.

- What are the consequences? How might this characteristic or practice impede your board's performance and contributions? What are the implications?

- Why does your board have this characteristic or engage in this practice? What are the reasons for it?

- How difficult would it be to change? What are the barriers to doing so?

Select from the lowest-rated characteristics and practices that have the greatest impact on your board's performance and contributions, five or six that you feel may be the most susceptible to change. For each, rough out an initial action plan. The key questions are these:

- What is the objective? What would this particular characteristic or practice look like at its very best?

- What specific things must be done to transform a problematic characteristic or practice into an exemplary one? Be concrete and precise; note the actions, tasks, and activities that would be necessary.

- What process should be undertaken to ensure success? What are the required steps and their sequence? Options might be general discussion of the problematic characteristic or practice with your board; assignment to a committee for analysis and the development of recommendations (for example, drafting principles that could alter your board's governance practice); review by legal counsel; board discussion, deliberation, and vote.

- What barriers and problems might arise? How can they be eliminated, reduced, or circumvented?
- How will you know that success has been achieved?
- What must be done to ensure that the change sticks?

PRINCIPLE-BASED GOVERNANCE PRACTICE

Assessment and action planning can Identify and begin to address specific problems that compromise your board's performance and contributions. But over the long run, to get to great, your board's governance practice must be based on and driven by a set of principles. Such principles will focus your board's precious and very limited attention, time, and energy. When continuously and consistently applied, they will guide the way your board meets its obligations, fulfills its responsibilities, performs its roles, designs its structure, crafts its composition, and builds and maintains infrastructure.

Start thinking about the specific principles your board should formulate and adopt.

- Review the seventy-two principles and associated practices set forth in this book. Which ones does your board presently employ (even though it may not recognize or formally codify them)? Which ones are not employed? Why?
- Identify about a dozen principles that, if adopted, would have the greatest impact on improving your board's performance and contributions.
- Try your hand at drafting a handful of principles for your board; some illustrations are provided in Appendix C.

TEAMWORK

All organizational change begins in the mind, heart, and soul of a single individual. But for change to be initiated, take hold, and have an impact, the circle of understanding and action must be expanded from you to your board as a whole. Here are recommendations for getting started.

- Suggest that copies of this book be made available to all board members, and encourage them to read it. Your board must have a collective understanding of principle-based governance and best governance practice.

- Devote a portion of a board meeting to discussing the ideas presented here and how they might be adopted by your board to improve its performance and contributions. Talk frankly about the costs and benefits of implementing a principle-based approach in whole or in part. Decide whether to move ahead.

- Have all members complete the Checkups, compile the responses, and calculate average scores for each individual item and dimension; then produce a "whole board" spider diagram. (It is important that members of your board read this book prior to completing the Checkups. This guards against members employing totally different definitions of key concepts in making their assessments. For example, to effectively assess whether your board understands and discharges its fundamental obligation, as explained in Principle 3, members must employ the same definition of this term.)

- Form an ad-hoc committee to review the assessment results, and begin drafting an initial set of governing principles for your board. We recommend developing no more than about a dozen that focus on specific practices identified as most problematic and potentially transforming. Circulate the draft principles among board members, and solicit their feedback.

- Hold a board retreat to review assessment results, discuss and deliberate draft principles, and develop action plans for implementing each principle (see Box 9.1 for an illustration).

- Codify the principles, and distribute them to all board members.

- Assign the responsibility of facilitating your board's principle-based approach to governing to a committee that will draft additional principles;

Box 9.1. Principle-Based Governance Action Planning

Principle

Our board will guide and direct the organization, on behalf of stakeholders, primarily through the formulation of policies regarding ends, executive performance, quality, finances, and governance. Where feasible and practical, action items and recommendations coming before the board for discussion and vote shall be framed as draft policies. Board policies will be codified and distributed employing a form specifically designed for this purpose. All board policies will be reviewed annually.

Action Planning Elements

- The CEO, board chair, and governance committee chair will read *Reinventing Your Board: A Step-by-Step Guide to Implementing Policy Governance*, by John Carver and Miriam Mayhew Carver, by (date).
- Chapters Two, Three, and Four and Appendix A of *Getting to Great* will be distributed to all board members by (date).
- A discussion of the policy governance approach will be held at the (date) board meeting; members will discuss, deliberate, and vote on whether to move forward with implementation.
- Follow-up and implementation planning will be assigned to the governance committee, which will

    Draft a policy codification form

    Conduct an audit of board meeting minutes for the past three years to identify "implicit policies"

    Draft an initial set of key policies for board discussion, deliberation, and vote
- A workshop on crafting policies at board meetings will be held by (date), and *CarverGuide*, "Basic Principles of Policy Governance," will be distributed to all board members.

bring them to your board for discussion, deliberation, and vote; and prepare action plans for ensuring their effective implementation.

- Annually assess whether your board is really governing on the basis of the principles it has adopted and the extent to which each principle results in better performance and greater contributions.

THE CONUNDRUM OF CHANGE

You've probably seen it happen numerous times: a change initiative begins with considerable fanfare; it is a great idea and makes sense, but it either fails to get off the ground or does not stick.

Inertia is a powerful force; all systems, including governance, are inherently resistant to change. In moving toward a principle-based approach, your board will be initiating very broad and deep change. Here are a few key recommendations.

Secure the "high ground" first. The board chair and CEO must be committed to principle-based governance. Other members can serve as catalysts, but without the full support of board leadership, it is highly unlikely that anything will happen. If you are the chair or CEO, you're on the way. If not, give them copies of this book, buy them dinner, start talking, and begin building a coalition for mounting change.

Build consensus regarding the need for change, and do not start the transformation process until you have it. "Happy systems do not change." Your board must be dissatisfied with the status quo; it must also develop a vision of the way things could be at their very best. The difference between "is" and "could be" provides the motivation for change. Discussing the principles and practices presented here, combined with a candid assessment of your board, is the point of departure.

Most boards are mired in an activity trap where the routine overwhelms the nonroutine. Their time is limited, and they spend so much of it actually governing, there is little energy left for improving how they govern. *For your board to mount a transformation, it must extricate itself from this trap.* You will have to step back from the routine, get out of the "way things have

Box 9.2. Trading Change

One of the best and most practical books we've read on this topic is *Leading Change* by John Kotter (Boston: Harvard Business School Press, 1996). He also wrote a companion article titled "Leading Change: Why Transformation Efforts Fail" (*Harvard Business Review*, Mar.-Apr. 1995). We recommend both.

Kotter argues that transformational efforts that seek to produce significant change often fail because of eight common errors:

- Too much complacency
- Not creating a powerful guiding coalition
- Underestimating the need for a precise and empowering vision of what things could and should be like
- Dramatically undercommunicating the need for change and the organization's vision
- Not removing obvious obstacles early in the process
- Not producing short-term wins
- Declaring victory too soon
- Neglecting to firmly anchor changes in the system's culture

He then proposes sets of strategies for overcoming these barriers.

---

always been done" box, and find the time necessary to design and implement new systems and procedures. There are no easy paths here, but finding time to do the additional work of transformation is critical. Do an audit of your board's activities (in general and particularly at its meetings). Identify things your board does that are irrelevant and inconsequential. Stop doing them, and use the time to engineer governance improvement initiatives. We have found that scheduling a series of half-day-long "miniretreats" over a year is one of the best ways to focus a board's attention on developing, adopting, and implementing governing principles and best practices.

Be realistic. Transforming a board is like remodeling a house. It is a disruptive process requiring considerable effort; you will go down some "blind alleys," and a number of difficulties will be encountered along the way.

Start small and keep at it. Principle-based governance can (and in our judgment should) be implemented incrementally. Indeed, the desire to radically change the culture of your board totally, by implementing a full set of principles across all dimensions of governance at one time, is probably doomed to failure. Our recommendation is to develop and implement focused sets of principles in waves. Begin with the basics, and become increasingly sophisticated, refined, and comprehensive over time.

Expect conflict. Engaging in increasingly explicit and precise discussions about how your board should govern will raise issues that were unrecognized, unclear, or ignored. Problem clarity always precipitates conflict regarding potential solutions. Such conflict (around ideas rather than personalities) should be embraced as a way to build energy and stimulate creativity.

Celebrate initial victories. Change initiatives are sustained through a series of small wins. Recognizing and celebrating short-term results provides evidence that the effort is worthwhile, undermines cynics and resisters, and builds motivation and momentum for the long run.

There is a positive, systematic, and ongoing association between governance quality and organizational success. Your board can make a difference on behalf of stakeholders and add real value. Or it can rob the organization of its potential. Which type of board will yours be?

APPENDIX A

SAMPLE BOARD POLICIES

ENDS

- Strategies are management's means for accomplishing organizational goals and the vision on behalf of stakeholders. The task of devising organizational strategies is delegated to management. At least two months prior to the start of the fiscal year, management must submit its key strategies to our board. Each strategy must be explicitly linked to one or more board-formulated goals. In addition, a rationale must be given that succinctly describes how pursuing the particular strategy will lead to accomplishing the goal or goals to which it is linked and the vision.

EXECUTIVE PERFORMANCE

- The CEO is the agent of our board and its only direct report. The CEO is delegated full authority for conducting the organization's affairs (including formulating strategies and managing its operations), constrained only by our board's policies and decisions, and subject to its oversight.

- The CEO is prohibited from authorizing, without prior board approval, individual capital expenditures exceeding $XX,XXX, expenditures for improvement in facilities exceeding $XX,XXX per project, leases exceeding $XXX,XXX in total value, expenditures for new programs and or programmatic enhancements exceeding $XX,XXX per year, and contracts for the purchase of services exceeding $XX,XXX.

QUALITY

- Management is directed to retain a consulting firm to conduct a periodic assessment (employing precise quantitative measures across multiple dimensions) of patient satisfaction and the extent to which the organization's services meet their needs, employee satisfaction, and medical staff satisfaction. Findings should be trended, compared to those of similar organizations, or benchmarked. Results of the assessment, in addition to management plans for correcting any deficiencies, should be presented to the board at least annually.

FINANCES

- The CEO is directed to design and implement, by (date), a compliance program to ensure that violations of applicable law and regulations by the organization's employees and agents are prevented, detected, reported, and corrected. An annual audit should be conducted with a report submitted to the board regarding how well the organization is complying with its legal and ethical obligations. This report should outline any recommended changes.

BOARD EFFECTIVENESS AND EFFICIENCY

- Policies of our board regarding its functioning, structure, composition, and infrastructure can be found in the bylaws. These bylaws supersede all policies formulated by our board regarding its own activities.

- Members of the board appointed ex officio have the same fiduciary duties as outside directors: to represent the interests of the organization's stakeholders as a general class. That is, ex officio members are appointed to our board because they bring valuable expertise, experience, and perspectives; they are not appointed to represent the special interests of a particular stakeholder group.

- Each board member shall exercise good faith and best efforts to fulfill his or her duties. Each board member will be held to a strict rule of loyalty, honesty, and fair dealing; no board member shall use his or her position or knowledge gained from it in a manner that would create a material conflict of interest or the appearance of such. In all matters affecting the organization, each board member shall act exclusively on behalf of stakeholder interests. No board member shall accept any material compensation, gift, or other favor that could influence or appear to influence his or her actions or decisions in the performance of his or her role. Each member, by completing our board's annual conflict-of-interest questionnaire, shall disclose any employment, activity, investment, or other interests that could compromise or conflict with the interests of the organization and its stakeholders. Each board member shall immediately disclose to the chair potential material conflicts when they arise. A member shall recuse himself or herself from any discussion, deliberation, or vote in which he or she has a material conflict of interest. No member shall claim the status of an agent of the organization unless specifically authorized to do so by the board.

SAMPLE
COMMITTEE
CHARTERS

EXECUTIVE COMMITTEE

The executive committee acts for our board in emergencies (when a quorum cannot be convened) and provides support to the chair in leading and planning the organization's governance. Its functions include the following:

- Developing, managing, and overseeing the board's budget
- Directing and overseeing staff allocated to our board
- Providing advice and counsel to the chairperson in appointing committee chairs and members
- Establishing ad hoc committees and appointing their members
- Drafting annual governance objectives and the work plan for our board's deliberation and approval
- Setting the agenda of board meetings
- Reviewing and making recommendations to our board regarding removal of members in midterm
- Providing advice and counsel to the chair regarding ways to enhance board performance and contributions
- Serving as a sounding board for the CEO regarding issues he or she may want to bring before it
- When the need arises, serving as our board's CEO search committee
- Undertaking other tasks as assigned by the board chair

COMMITTEE ON ENDS

The committee on ends helps our board formulate policies, make decisions, and oversee the organization's ends (vision, goals, and strategies) and advance and protect stakeholder interests. Its functions include the following:

- Helping our board undertake periodic analyses of key stakeholders, including their interests, needs, and expectations

- Formulating or reformulating a draft organizational vision for board deliberation and action

- Formulating or reformulating draft organizational goals for board deliberation and action

- Engaging annually in a preliminary assessment of the extent to which management strategies are aligned with the board-formulated vision and key goals and submitting this assessment to our board for deliberation and action

- Recommending quantitative measures to be employed by the board in monitoring and assessing whether the organization's vision is being fulfilled, goals are being accomplished, and key strategies are being effectively pursued

- Drafting policies regarding organizational ends and submitting them to our board for deliberation and action

- Reviewing proposals regarding organizational ends submitted by management and submitting them (with comments and recommendations) to our board for deliberation and action

- Preparing drafts of decisions regarding organizational ends that must be made by our board

- Undertaking an annual review and assessment of all board policies and decisions regarding organizational ends

- Performing other tasks dealing with organizational ends as assigned by our board

COMMITTEE ON EXECUTIVE PERFORMANCE

The committee helps our board formulate policies, make decisions, and engage in oversight to ensure high levels of executive performance. Its functions include the following:

- Conducting a semiannual review of the CEO succession plan and submitting recommendations to our board regarding needed alterations
- Undertaking an annual review of the CEO's employment contract
- Working with the CEO to formulate annual personal performance expectations and submitting them to our board for deliberation and approval
- On behalf of our board, undertaking an assessment of the CEO's performance, engaging in action planning with the CEO to improve his or her performance, and submitting this assessment and recommendations for adjustments in compensation to our board for deliberation and approval
- Conducting a semiannual review of our board's CEO assessment process and making recommendations for needed alterations
- Drafting policies regarding executive management performance and forwarding them to the board for deliberation and action
- Reviewing and analyzing proposals regarding executive management performance and submitting them to our board for deliberation and action
- Drafting decisions regarding executive management performance that must be made by our board
- Recommending quantitative measures to be employed by our board in assessing the CEO's performance
- Undertaking an annual assessment of all board policies and decisions regarding CEO performance
- Performing other tasks related to the enhancement of executive management performance as assigned by our board

QUALITY COMMITTEE

The quality committee assists our board by credentialing members of the medical staff and formulating policies, making decisions, and engaging in oversight that ensures high levels of quality and customer satisfaction. Its functions include the following:

- Working with management to undertake an annual analysis of patient or customer needs and the extent to which the organization is meeting them and submitting this assessment to our board for review

- On a case-by-case basis, fully, rigorously, and carefully reviewing recommendations of the medical staff executive committee regarding the appointment, reappointment, and privilege delineation of physicians and submitting its recommendations to our board for review and action

- Undertaking an annual assessment of the adequacy of the organization's quality monitoring and management systems and submitting recommendations to our board for its deliberation and action

- Annually reviewing management's plans for continuously improving quality and submitting its analysis and recommendations to our board for discussion and approval

- Drafting policies regarding quality and submitting them to our board for deliberation and action

- Reviewing management proposals regarding quality and submitting them to our board for deliberation and action

- Drafting decisions regarding quality that must be made by our board

- Recommending quantitative measures to be employed by our board in assessing quality

- Conducting a quarterly review of quality measures and submitting an analysis to our board for deliberation and action

- Undertaking an annual assessment of all board policies and decisions regarding quality

- Performing other tasks related to quality as assigned by our board

FINANCE COMMITTEE

The finance committee assists our board in formulating policies, making decisions, and engaging in oversight that ensures the organization's financial health. Its functions include the following:

- Annually forming a subcommittee to oversee the audit and reviewing the auditor's opinion and management letter prior to deliberation and action by our board

- Reviewing all proposals from management regarding operational and capital expenditures that exceed board-preapproved authorization limits and submitting recommendations to our board for deliberation and action

- Annually submitting a memo to our board reviewing and assessing the organization's overall financial states and health

- Serving as the point of first contact for the internal auditor's interaction with our board regarding any concerns he or she may wish to raise regarding appropriate use and distribution of funds

- Drafting policies regarding finances and submitting them to our board for deliberation and action

- Reviewing and analyzing proposals made by management regarding finances and submitting them to our board for deliberation and action

- Drafting decisions regarding finances that must be made by our board

- Recommending quantitative measures to be employed by our board in assessing the organization's financial health

- Conducting a quarterly review of financial measures and submitting an analysis to our board for deliberation and action

- Undertaking an annual assessment of all board policies and decisions regarding finances

- Performing other tasks related to the organization's financial health as assigned by our board

GOVERNANCE COMMITTEE

The governance committee helps our board improve its own functioning, structure, composition, and infrastructure. Its functions include the following:

- Directing and overseeing the semiannual assessment of our board, board committees, and individual board members; reviewing these assessments; and making recommendations to the board regarding ways in which its performance and contributions can be enhanced

- Planning the annual board retreat

- Directing and overseeing our board's continuing education and development activities

- Assessing the qualifications of individuals to assume board seats and submitting nominations to our board

- Designing our board's new-member orientation process and periodically assessing it

- Drafting policies regarding governance performance and submitting them to our board for deliberation and action

- Drafting decisions regarding governance performance and submitting them to our board for deliberation and action

- Recommending quantitative measures to be employed by our board in assessing governance performance and contributions

- Conducting an annual review of governance performance measures and submitting an analysis to our board for deliberation and action

- Undertaking an annual assessment of all board policies and decisions regarding governance performance

- Performing other tasks related to governance and contributions as assigned by our board

APPENDIX C

SAMPLE GOVERNANCE PRINCIPLES

Our board's governance practice is principle-based. These principles are continuously and consistently applied to the way our board meets its obligations, fulfills its responsibilities, performs its roles, designs its structure, crafts its composition, and creates and maintains its infrastructure. These principles are thoroughly reviewed annually and modified if necessary.

1. Our organization exists to benefit its stakeholders. Our board's purpose, and overarching obligation, is to ensure that stakeholder interests are protected and advanced and that the organization's resources and capacities are effectively and efficiently deployed.

2. At least every three years, our board conducts a stakeholder analysis identifying key stakeholder groups and analyzing and understanding their needs, interests, and expectations.

3. All issues coming before our board are discussed, deliberated, and acted on from a stakeholder perspective.

4. It is the duty of each board member to balance the needs and expectations of all stakeholders, not to advocate narrow interests or represent specific interest groups.

5. Our board formulates our organization's vision on behalf of stakeholders, based on an analysis of their needs, interests, and expectations. The vision is an explicit, precise, fine-grained, and empowering image of what

our organization should become, in the future, at its very best; it denotes the organization's core purposes and values. The vision is reviewed by our board semiannually and modified if necessary.

6. Our board specifies the organization's key goals, the most important things the organization must accomplish in order to fulfill the vision. Each year, our board: formulates key goals and reviews and modifies them if necessary; employing explicit criteria, it assesses the extent they are being accomplished.

7. Annually, our board specifies its most important performance expectations of the CEO.

8. Employing explicit criteria and a formal process, our board evaluates the CEO's performance annually in terms of the extent to which stakeholder needs and expectations are being met, the vision is being fulfilled, key goals are being achieved, strategies are being effectively pursued, key financial performance and outcome objectives are being attained, and the CEO's personal performance expectations are being met.

9. Employing explicit criteria and based on a valid methodology, the CEO reports to our board annually regarding the quality of care provided in and by the organization and patient or customer satisfaction.

10. Annually, our board formulates a set of precise financial objectives for the organization.

11. Board committees develop annual objectives and work plans. They are reviewed and approved by the executive committee.

12. Member service on our board is limited to no more than three successive terms of three years each. The renewal of a member's term is not automatic but rather based on an assessment of his or her performance and contributions in addition to organizational and board needs.

13. The performance and contribution of each board member are assessed prior to the end of his or her term. This assessment is employed by the executive committee to counsel the member regarding his or her development and to determine if he or she should be renominated for a new term.

14. Each year, a set of board goals is developed specifying the most important things our board must accomplish. The degree to which these goals have been achieved is assessed annually.

APPENDIX D

RESOURCES

BOOKS

Board Work: Governing Health Care Organizations, by Dennis D. Pointer and James E. Orlikoff (San Francisco: Jossey-Bass, 1999)

Boards That Make a Difference: A New Design for Leadership in Nonprofit and Public Organizations, by John Carver (San Francisco: Jossey-Bass, 1997)

The Effective Board of Trustees, by Richard P. Chait, Thomas P. Holland, and Barbara E. Taylor (Westport, Conn.: Oryx Press, 1993)

Governing Boards: Their Nurture and Nature, by Cyril O. Houle (San Francisco: Jossey-Bass, 1989)

Reinventing Your Board: A Step-by-Step Guide to Implementing Policy Governance, by John Carver and Miriam Mayhew Carver (San Francisco: Jossey-Bass, 1997)

ARTICLES

"Charting the Territory of Nonprofit Boards," by Richard P. Chait and Barbara E. Taylor (*Harvard Business Review,* Jan. 1989)

"The New Work of the Nonprofit Board," by Barbara E. Taylor and colleagues (*Harvard Business Review,* Sept.-Oct. 1996)

"Really Governing: What Type of Work Should Your Board Be Doing?" by Dennis D. Pointer and Charles M. Ewell (*Hospital and Health Services Administration,* May-June 1995)

"Trouble in the Board Room: The Seven Deadly Sins of Ineffective Governance," by James E. Orlikoff (*Healthcare Forum Journal,* May-June 1997)

WEB SITES

American Governance and Leadership Group, www.american governance.com

Board of Directors Network, www.boarddirectorsnetwork.org

Business Roundtable, www.brtable.org

California Public Employees Retirement System, www.calpers.org

Conference Board, www.conference-board.org

Corporate Directors' Forum, www.directorsforum.com

Corporate Library, www.thecorporatelibrary.net

Encyclopedia of Corporate Governance, www.encycogov.com

Internet Nonprofit Center, www.nonprofits.org

National Association of Corporate Directors, www.nacdonline.org

National Center for Nonprofit Boards, www.boardsource.org

INDEX

Hospitals: Catholic, *23*, *36*; short-term, *21*, *36*, *38*; and structure, 99, *100*

Houle, C. O., 191

How to Make Meetings Work! The New Interaction Method (Doyle and Straus), *152*

How to Run a Successful Meeting—in Half the Time (Frank), *152*

Huston, J., *116*

I

Illegal or unethical behavior, 49

Incentive compensation, 48

Incremental change, 178

Indicators: and assessment, 59, *75*; examples of, *60*; financial, types of, 67–68; of overall board fitness, 170; and oversight, 83–84, *85*, 86, 87, 88, 101; quality, *60*

Individuality and structure design, 97

Information items, 149

Infrastructure: checkup on, 165–166; definition of, 11; designing, need for, 13; expenditures on, areas of, 141–142; getting started on, 166–167; and meeting obligations, *12*; overview of, 141; and policy, *76*; principles on, 141–164; scoring on, diagramming, 170, *171*; and structure, 97; summary on, *8*. *See also* Board effectiveness, efficiency, and creativity

Insider board members, 131–132

Insurance company, captive liability, *100*

Intentional structure design, 97

Interim CEO appointees, 44–45

Interlocking board membership, 100, *102*

Internal (management) boards, 100, *102*

Internal Revenue Service (IRS), compensation and, 48–49

Internet Nonprofit Center, 192

J

Job descriptions: for board chair, 156, 157–158, 159; for board coordinators, *143*; for board members, opinions of, 123

K

Kehoe, K. R., *152*

Kieffer, G. D., *152*

Kotter, J., *177*

L

Lake metaphor, *10*

Large boards, disadvantages of, 103–104

Leadership role, 156

Leading Change (Kotter), *177*

"Leading Change: Why Transformation Efforts Fail" (Kotter), *177*

Legal fiduciary duty: and advisory boards, 106; of care in discharging responsibilities, 24, 25–26, 71; and committees, 108; of loyalty to stakeholders, 23–24, *25*, 71

Legal requirements for subsidiaries, 99

Liquidity, 68

Listening and talking, time spent on, 88, *89*, 151, *152*, 163–164

Low performance, assessment of, 171–172

Loyalty to stakeholders, legal fiduciary duty of, 23–24, *25*, 71

M

Magazines and newsletters, subscribing to, 160

Management: delegating to, 39–40, 65, 66–67; role of, in formulating vision, 37

Management leaders, interacting with, during retreats, 163

Management staff, responsibility for, 43

Management technology, 1, 2

Management work, distinguishing, from governance work, *40*, 43, 67

Mapping, 105, *106*

Meals: and meetings, 145; and retreats, 163

Means and end, 18

Medical groups and structure, 99, *100*

Medical staff: as board members, 131, 136; and physician credentialing, *56*, 57, 58

Medical staff office, *56*

Meeting time, allocation of: to addressing principles, 174; to listening and talking, 151, *152*; to meeting assessment, 154; planning and managing, 145, *146–148*, 149, 150; to questions and discussions, 153; to role-related activity, 88, *89*

Meetings: assessment of, 154; attendance at, increasing, 135; managing and conducting, 144, 145, 150–155

Meetings That Work! A Practical Guide to Shorter and More Productive Meetings (Chang and Kehoe), *152*

Mentoring, 123

Metaphors depicting challenges of governance, *10*

Methods, focus on, 76, 77

Minimalism and committee design, 109

Miniretreats, 177

Minutes, recording, 153–154, *155*

Mirror boards, 100, *102*

Mirroring stakeholder characteristics, 129–130

Mission and vision, difference between, *34*

Monitoring, 58, 67, 84, *85*, 86. *See also* Oversight

N

National Association of Corporate Directors, *162*, 192

National Center for Nonprofit Boards, *162*, 192

"New Work of the Nonprofit Board, The" (Taylor), 191

Nomination of board chairs, *158*

Nonrepresentational composition, 128–130

O

Objectives, annual, development of, 142, 144. *See also* Financial objectives

Obligations: checkup on, 28–29; definition of, 11; getting started on, 29; key factors in meeting, *12*; principles on, 17–19, 21–28; reinforcing, in meetings, 151; responsibilities and, 26, *27*; roles

and, 27; scoring on, diagramming, *171*; summary on, *5*

Off-site outpatient surgery program, quality of, differing perspectives on, *54*

On the Origin of Species (Darwin), 4

Operations expenditures for boards, 142

Opportunity costs, reimbursement for, 135

Organization, defining, 18

Organizational advocates, serving as, 71, 72, 106

Organizational ends (destination). *See* Ends

Organizational performance, 11

Orientation for new board members, 120–123, 159

Orlikoff, J. E., 8, *55*, *161*, 192

Oversight: and agendas, *147–148*; dashboards for, 82, 86–87; in decentralized structure, *106*; defined, 73; delegating and, 83; dividing responsibility for, *107*; and graphical approach to reporting, 87–88; and obligations, 27; by parent boards, 101, 103; principles on, 82–88, *89*; process of, 83–84, *85–86*. *See also* Monitoring

Oversight committees, 103

P

Parent boards: and appointing boards, 115; and charting structure, *100*; choosing by, between centralized and decentralized structure, 98–99; oversight by, 101, 103; roles and responsibilities of, specifying, 105, *106*, *107*; structural options for, 100, *102*; and structure, 95

Partnership relationship aspect, 130

Patient care, quality of. *See Quality entries*

Performance. *See* Board performance; Executive performance; Financial performance; Organizational performance

Per-meeting fees, 135–136

Personal contributions, making, 71

Physician leaders, interacting with, during retreats, 163

Physicians: as board members, 131, 136; credentialing, 55–58, *75*